Nursing Care Planning

made Incredibly Easy!

Third Edition

Nursing Care Planning

made
Incredibly
Easy!®

Third Edition

Clinical Editor
Theresa Capriotti, DO, MSN, CRNP, RN
Clinical Associate Professor
Villanova University College of Nursing
Villanova, Pennsylvania

. Wolters Kluwer

Philadelphia • Baltimore • New York • London
Buenos Aires • Hong Kong • Sydney • Tokyo

Acquisitions Editor: Nicole Dernoski
Developmental Editor: Maria M. McAvey
Editorial Coordinator: Jennifer DiRicco
Editorial Assistant: Kathryn Leyendecker
Production Project Manager: Marian Bellus
Design Coordinator: Elaine Kasmer
Manufacturing Coordinator: Kathleen Brown
Marketing Manager: Linda Wetmore
Prepress Vendor: SPi Global

3rd edition

Library of Congress Cataloging-in-Publication Data
Names: Capriotti, Theresa, editor.
Title: Nursing care planning made incredibly easy! / clinical editor, Theresa Capriotti.
Description: 3rd edition. | Philadelphia : Wolters Kluwer, [2018] | Includes bibliographical references and index.
Identifiers: LCCN 2017039562 | ISBN 9781496382566
Subjects: | MESH: Nursing Process | Patient Care Planning | Handbooks | Examination Questions
Classification: LCC RT41 | NLM WY 49 | DDC 610.73—dc23 LC record available at https://lccn.loc.gov/2017039562

LWW.com

Dedication

This book is dedicated to my beloved grandson, Ethan Vincent Wolinsky. And to Rocco, Gigi, and Puccini, my most faithful friends.

Teri Capriotti

Contributors

Louise A. Aurilio, PhD, RN-BC, NE-BC
Professor Emeritus
Nursing Department
Youngstown State University
Youngstown, Ohio

Carol A. Blakeman, MSN, ARNP
Senior Professor
College of Central Florida, Health
    Sciences
Ocala, Florida

Cheryl Brady, MSN, CNE
Nursing Faculty
College of Nursing
Kent State University
Salem, Ohio

Linda Carman Copel, RN, PhD, CS, DAPA
Professor
Villanova University
Villanova, Pennsylvania

Susan B. Dickey, RN, PhD
Associate Professor
Department of Nursing
College of Public Health
Temple University
Philadelphia, Pennsylvania

Valerie Flattes, APRN, MS, ANP-BC
Assistant Professor, Clinical
College of Nursing
University of Utah
Salt Lake City, Utah

Marilyn Little, APRN, PP
APRN Prescriber
Valley Mental Health
West Valley City, Utah

Bette Mariani, RNC-MNN, MSN
Assistant Professor of Nursing
College of Nursing
Villanova University
Villanova, Pennsylvania

Jill Morsbach, MSN, RNC-MNN
Assistant Professor
School of Nursing & Health Professions
Missouri Western State University
St. Joseph, Missouri

Mary L. Nesbitt, BSN, MAN, RNC
Associate Professor of Nursing
William Carey University
Biloxi, Mississippi

Noel C. Piano, RN, MS
Instructor and Program Director
Lafayette School of Practical Nursing
Williamsburg, Virginia

Marilyn D. Sellers, MSN, FNP-BC, RN-BC
Family Nurse Practitioner
Compensation and Pension Department
WJ Dorn VAMC
Columbia, South Carolina

Previous Edition Contributors

Louise A. Aurilio, PhD, RN-BC, NE-BC

Susan Barnason, PhD, RN, CEN, CCRN, CS

Carol A. Blakeman, MSN, ARNP

Cheryl Brady, MSN, CNE

Natalie C. Burkhalter, RN, MSN, FNP, ACNP, CCRN

Anita L. Caroll, EdD, MSN, RN

Michael A. Carter, DNSc, FAAN, APRN-BC

Karen Demzien Connors, MSN, CNE

Linda Carman Copel, RN, PhD, CS, DAPA

Patricia D. Coyne, RNC-MNN, MS, MPA

Susan B. Dickey, RN, PhD

Gloria F. Donnelly, PhD, RN, FAAN

Caroline Dorsen, MSN, APRN, BC, FNP

Valerie Flattes, APRN, MS, ANP-BC

Stephen Gilliam, PhD, FNP, APRN-BC

Margaret Mary Hansen, EdD, MSN, RN, NI Certificate

Kathy Henley Haugh, PhD, RN

Janice J. Hoffman, PhD, RN, CCRN

Leslie Holmes, RN, MSN

Karla R. Jones, MS, RN

Marilyn Little, APRN, PP

Kay Luft, RN, MN, CNE, CCRN

Marilyn K. Miller, MSN, RN

Jill Morsbach, RNC-MNN, MSN

Judith A. Murphy, BSN, RN

Holly Myers, MSN, RN

Mary L. Nesbitt, BSN, MAN, RNC

Kristie S. Nix, EdD, RN

Tracy Stephens Patil, MSN, RN

Linda Honan Pellico, PhD, MSN, APRN

Theresa Petersen, MSN, APRN

Ellen Pfadt, PhD(C), RN

Noel C. Piano, RN, MS

Deborah A. Raines, PhD, RN, ANEF

N. Darlene Rainwater, RN, MSN

Darlene Samuelson, RN, BS, MEd, MSN

Patricia J. Sands, RN, MSN-PNP, CPNP-PC, CEN

Marilyn D. Sellers, MSN, FNP-BC, RN-BC

Michele Woodbeck, MS, RN

Susan L. Woods, PhD, RN, FAAN, FAHA

Denise R. York, RNC, CNS, MS, MEd

Foreword

The 2010 Institute of Medicine (IOM) Report, "The Future of Nursing," clearly articulates the need for our profession to lead change and advance the health of all populations. This position paper states that the nursing education system must be improved to ensure the safe delivery of patient-centered care across life's transitions, from conception to death. To assure this professional mandate, the IOM Report stresses that nurses must be prepared to practice to the full extent of their education and training. Furthermore, nurses should be full partners with physicians and other health care professionals in redesigning the health care delivery system.

Nursing's unique contribution to this partnership and to patient care and outcomes is the individualized nursing plan of care. This third edition of *Nursing Care Planning Made Incredibly Easy* offers novice nurses and students an updated global positioning–oriented navigation system for how to articulate and demonstrate the *value* that nursing practice brings to patient outcomes. This book describes the importance of the nursing process and of mastering a concept map framework to better implement the nursing process. The subsequent plan of care evolves naturally as an extension of this process, and the use of electronic medical records and other technological advancements helps ensure that all members of the nursing team have access to the same information to address patient and family needs when delivering care.

In Part I, you'll find a discussion of three classification systems, which have been updated for this edition: *NANDA-I*, which defines standardized nursing diagnoses; *NOC*, which identifies patient outcomes; and NIC, which lists nursing care interventions that align with NANDA-I and NOC. In Part II, you'll see how specific nursing diagnoses relate to common medical-surgical, psychiatric, maternal-neonatal, and pediatric medical diagnoses. Additionally, you'll have online access to 166 customizable care plans covering every nursing specialty, including new plans for gastric bypass, preterm labor, and cerebral palsy.

As you read through this text, look for these eye-catching logos to focus your attention on essential information:

 Under construction offers sample concept maps and care plan components, plus tips for making care plans specific and individualized.

 Weighing the evidence provides information on the latest evidence-based standards of care used in the sample care plans.

Teacher knows best imparts important reminders from Instructor Joy to help you understand how to apply content.

Memory jogger mnemonic devices help you to remember key concepts and content.

Although computerized care plans are becoming more common in practice, keep in mind that they are only a *tool* and a *guide* to help you think critically about the individualized care needed by your patients and their families. Take the time to learn and understand NANDA diagnoses, NOC, and NIC, as these standards will surely become mainstays in our practice for providing quality, cost-saving outcomes. And remember, the basis of a successful nursing practice begins with you, the nurse, and your understanding that each patient is an individual with unique needs. When caring for each patient, begin by building a concept map and using the nursing process to develop a nursing diagnosis, realistic and achievable outcomes, and individualized interventions; then, assess and reassess as you provide care. Follow this approach throughout your budding career, and the vision of the "Future of Nursing" will be your reality.

Victoria L. Rich, PhD, RN, FAAN
Chief Nurse Executive
Hospital of the University of Pennsylvania
Philadelphia, Pennsylvania

Contents

Part I

Care planning using the nursing process

Chapter 1

Introduction to care planning

Just the facts

In this chapter, you'll learn:
- ◆ the benefits of using the nursing process
- ◆ the role of the nursing process in planning patient care
- ◆ ways in which the nursing process promotes critical thinking
- ◆ fundamentals of concept mapping and its uses in care planning.

A look at care planning

A crucial component of nursing care, a care plan (*also referred to as a plan of care*) serves as a road map that guides all health care team members involved in a patient's care. Developing a plan of care allows a nurse to identify a patient's problems and select interventions that will help solve or minimize these problems and contribute to safe, quality patient care.

The great communicator

The care plan also communicates vital patient information to the entire interprofessional health care team. It contains detailed instructions for achieving the goals established for the patient.

Understanding the nursing process

Effective care planning results from the nursing process—a deliberate, systematic process that takes a problem-solving approach to nursing care. Using the nursing process establishes the foundation for clinical reasoning as required by National Practice Standards.

Analyze, address, implement, evaluate

The cornerstone of clinical nursing, the nursing process gives you a structure for applying your knowledge and skills in an organized, goal-oriented way. It helps you think critically, solve problems, and make care decisions tailored to each patient's individual needs.

The nursing process requires you to systematically analyze patient data, make inferences, draw conclusions about patient

Think of a care plan as a map that helps the health care team stay on course when it comes to patient care.

problems, devise a care plan to address those problems, implement the plan, evaluate the plan's effectiveness, and revise the plan if necessary. This practice is critical to ensuring safe, quality care.

Oh, the humanity

The nursing process is holistic and humanistic. It addresses the human response to medical conditions—how these conditions affect the patient's life. To use it correctly, you must consider not just the patient's physical, mental, and emotional status but also the patient's interests, lifestyle, values, beliefs, and ethnic, religious, and cultural background.

Advantages of the nursing process

When used effectively, the nursing process offers many advantages:
- It provides an organized framework for nursing care delivery.
- It is patient centered, helping to ensure that your patient's health problems and his/her response to them are the focus of care.
- It enables you to individualize care for each patient.
- It promotes the patient's participation in care, encourages independence and compliance, and gives the patient a greater sense of control—important factors in a positive health outcome. (See *Putting the "P" in planning*.)
- It improves communication by providing you and other interprofessional team health care providers with a common list of the patient's recognized health problems.
- It promotes accountability for nursing activities based on evaluation, which in turn promotes quality assurance.
- It promotes critical thinking and forms the foundation for decision making and problem solving.
- It is outcome-focused and encourages the evaluation of results.
- It minimizes errors and omissions in care planning and promotes a competent level of care.

Teacher knows best

Putting the "P" in planning

Always remember to include the "P"—the patient—in planning. Ask for your patient's input when identifying problems, establishing outcomes, and formulating interventions. Doing this validates the importance of the patient and motivates him/her to participate in their own health care and adhere to the care plan. It also gives the patient a greater sense of control, which promotes personal responsibility and strengthens the patient's commitment to working toward the established goals.

Basis for the nursing process

The nursing process is based on the scientific method of problem solving, which involves:

- stating the problem or risk for a problem that you observed
- forming a hypothesis about the solution to the problem ("if-then" statements)
- developing a method to test the hypothesis
- collecting the test data
- analyzing the data
- drawing conclusions about the hypothesis.

A scientific fact

Most people use the scientific method instinctively, without being aware they're doing it. Simply picking out which pair of shoes best complements your favorite outfit is an exercise in the scientific method. So if you're familiar with the scientific process, the nursing process probably seems familiar.

Picking out shoes is scientific? I knew there was a good reason it took me so long—I just always thought it was all of the shoes.

Nursing process steps

The nursing process encompasses five steps:

1. assessment
2. nursing diagnosis
3. planning
4. implementation
5. evaluation.

Following these steps systematically in this order enables you to organize and prioritize patient care—especially critical for the novice nursing student. It also helps ensure that you don't skip or overlook important information. (See *Just how many steps are there?* [page 6].)

When used correctly, the nursing process ensures that the care plan is revised when new problems arise or patient outcomes remain unmet. It also allows the care plan to be discontinued when patient outcomes have been met.

Domino effect

Although the five nursing process steps are sequential, they also are continuous and interconnected. For instance, when performing an intervention, such as changing your patient's dressing, you should also be assessing his/her skin. (See *The nursing process: An unbroken circle.*)

Just how many steps are there?

Nurses are accountable for maintaining national practice standards, such as those set by the American Nurses Association (ANA). These standards state that "the nursing process encompasses all significant actions taken by registered nurses and forms the foundation for decision-making." However, the number of nursing process steps into which this definition translates varies.

The initial definition of the nursing process from the 1950s listed only three steps: assessment, planning, and evaluation. However, the ANA cites six steps in the nursing process:

- assessment
- nursing diagnosis
- outcome identification
- planning
- implementation
- evaluation.

Many authors and instructors have found it useful to combine outcome identification into the planning step because it's so closely allied to the choice of appropriate nursing interventions.

Remember that the nursing process guides all the nurse's *actions* and *decisions*, regardless of the number of steps cited.

What's more, these steps are interrelated, with each one influencing all the subsequent steps. For instance:

- Your assessment must be thorough and accurate so that you formulate the appropriate nursing diagnosis or problem list.
- The nursing diagnosis or problem list you formulate must be appropriate to ensure that you choose reasonable outcomes.
- The outcomes you identify must be appropriate so that you outline correct interventions.
- The interventions you choose must be appropriate so that your patient will make progress toward the outcomes you've established.

If you go astray during any step—say, by misinterpreting the assessment data—you can get back on track by reassessing the patient, evaluating his/her care plan, and revising the plan if necessary.

Assessment

The first step in the nursing process, assessment involves the systematic collection and recording of patient data. A comprehensive assessment gives you a wide-angle view of your patient's health problems, aiding in crucial decisions about quality patient care.

The nursing process: An unbroken circle

The nursing process is a progression of actions that continually recycle as patient problems and priorities change or resolve. In any specific task you do, more than one step may be involved.

Take for example...

When you initially assess a new patient's lungs, you begin the process of determining if the patient has any actual or potential problems related to respiratory function. In addition to assessing respiratory function, you can assess the skin integrity on the patient's chest and back.

The next time you assess the patient's lungs, you can evaluate whether your intervention to teach the patient use of an incentive spirometer was effective in keeping his/her lungs clear. When you do this, however, you notice that the patient's apical heartbeat is rapid and irregular—a change from your initial *assessment*. Now you quickly:

• conclude that the spirometry has been effective so far (*evaluation*)

• identify that the patient is at risk for decreased cardiac tissue perfusion (*nursing diagnosis*)

• identify that the patient's heart rate should return to less than 100 beats/minute with a regular rhythm (*planning expected outcomes*)

• determine that you should ask the patient how he or she is feeling to identify associated symptoms, check the patient's pulse oximetry to assess the need for supportive oxygen, obtain an immediate 12-lead electrocardiogram, and notify the health care practitioner of the change (*planning interventions*)

• put your devised plan into action (*implementation*).

Actual vs. Risk for nursing diagnoses

When formulating your patient's nursing diagnoses, you need to specify whether your patient has each problem or is at risk for developing it. Here's the distinction:

• If the patient has identifiable signs and symptoms that appear in all or most patients with the disorder, you should label the problem with an *actual* nursing diagnosis.

• If the patient has risk factors for a problem but doesn't have signs or symptoms, you should label the problem with a *Risk for* diagnosis.

Take impaired skin integrity, for example. If the patient has an open skin area, he/she has *actual* impaired skin integrity and the patient's diagnosis would be *Impaired skin integrity*. If he/she has no signs of skin breakdown but is bedbound and has bowel and bladder incontinence, he/she has predisposing factors that place the patient at risk for impaired skin integrity; therefore, the patient's nursing diagnosis would be *Risk for impaired skin integrity*.

Nursing diagnosis

The second step requires you to use your assessment data to formulate a problem list that will lead to nursing diagnoses—clinical judgments about the patient's response to an actual or potential health problem that nurses are legally permitted to manage. (See *Actual vs. Risk* for *nursing diagnoses*.) Remember, nursing diagnoses are different from medical diagnoses. (See *How nursing and medical diagnoses differ*.)

After the patient's problems or responses have been identified and reframed as nursing diagnoses, a quick review of the assessment findings and diagnoses can help you to correctly prioritize the most urgent needs of the patient.

Although both are important parts of patient care, medical diagnoses and nursing diagnoses are different.

Three's company

Each nursing diagnosis has three components:
• label—an actual or potential problem that nursing care can affect
• related factors—factors that may precede, contribute to, or be associated with the human response
• evidence—signs and symptoms that point to the nursing diagnosis.

Suppose, for instance, that your patient has constipation resulting from use of opioid analgesics for pain. You would formulate a nursing diagnosis of *Constipation related to use of opioid analgesics as evidenced by passage of hard, formed stools*.

How nursing and medical diagnoses differ

Practitioners such as doctors, nurse practitioners, and physician assistants diagnose and treat medical conditions related to anatomy, physiology, disease, or trauma. They formulate medical diagnoses that center on these medical diseases and conditions.

Nurses aren't licensed to diagnose medical diseases and conditions. Instead, they formulate nursing diagnoses that focus on how the patient responds to the medical disease or condition. Unlike medical diagnoses, nursing diagnoses are patient centered.

This case study will help you understand the difference between medical and nursing diagnoses.

Point, counterpoint
Mr. Mills is a 52-year-old man who was hospitalized after falling on a patch of ice and injuring his right hip. He's married and has two children, one of whom attends college. Mr. Mills works as a construction foreman; his wife is unemployed.

The practitioner's viewpoint
Here's how the practitioner sees the situation: Mr. Mills presents with pain in the right hip, a shortened right leg, and external rotation of the right hip after sustaining a fall on a patch of ice. The hip X-ray shows a well-defined intertrochanteric fracture of the right hip. The medical diagnosis is a *right hip fracture*. The medical plan is to proceed with open reduction and internal fixation of the hip.

The nurse's perspective
Here's how the nurse views the same patient information: Mr. Mills has pain in his right hip. He expresses an immediate concern about the need to urinate. He's also concerned about his job and lack of income during the recuperation period, when he won't be able to work. He says he has always been the breadwinner of his family, and he's worried that if he needs to be off work for a long time, he won't have the money to pay his son's college tuition. The initial nursing diagnoses for Mr. Mills are *Acute pain related to right hip fracture; Impaired urinary elimination related to inability to stand, pain, and voluntary retention; Anxiety related to financial concerns; and Risk for situational low self-esteem related to anticipated loss of roles as employee and family provider.*

The differences
The nurse focuses on Mr. Mills and his *responses* to the hip fracture. The nurse isn't licensed to treat the patient's hip fracture independently but can address problems stemming from his responses to the fracture, such as pain and discomfort, concern with urination, and the expected role change.

The nursing care plan should address Mr. Mills' pain management needs as well as include education about the indwelling urinary catheter that the nurse will place, a social service consult to address Mr. Mills' financial concerns, and assistance in working through his expected role changes.

One thing leads to another

Correctly identifying the problem and its cause is crucial to the next steps of the nursing process—planning and implementation.

Planning

During the planning stage of the nursing process, you:
- identify expected patient outcomes, or goals
- select nursing interventions designed to achieve these outcomes
- document the care plan, which becomes a permanent part of the patient's record and communicates the patient's needs to all health care providers who use the plan.

Here come the outcomes

For every nursing diagnosis, you must identify expected outcomes— measurable, patient-focused, time-specific goals the patient should reach as a result of the nursing interventions you've planned.

Outcomes derive from the nursing diagnosis. You must state them in terms of the patient's behavior. For example, if the patient has a nursing diagnosis of *Deficient knowledge (incision care)*, one reasonable outcome might be "Patient will verbalize precautions to take to prevent incision infection until healed."

Next in line—the interventions

Once you've identified the patient's problem or response and determined a reasonable outcome measurement, you can begin to list the steps that must be taken to reach that goal. Interventions are brief descriptions of specific actions. They should be based on the best evidence available documenting effectiveness and validity for achieving the desired outcome, and they should conform to appropriate standards of care.

Don't forget documentation. It's an important part of the process.

Don't forget to document

Always document the care plan so it's accessible to other health care team members. This communication provides crucial patient information to other interprofessional health care team members, promoting continuity of care.

Implementation

The next step in the nursing process is implementation, when you perform the actual interventions to help your patient reach the expected outcomes. But before carrying out these interventions, be sure to quickly reassess the patient to make sure that the interventions you've planned are still necessary. Patient situations can change rapidly, making some interventions inappropriate or unnecessary.

Throughout your nursing care, you'll need to evaluate the effectiveness of your interventions and make changes as needed. If you continue to implement ineffective interventions, you and your patient will lose valuable time. (See *Be pliable about care plans*.)

Evaluation

During the evaluation step of the nursing process, you:

- reassess the patient
- compare your findings with the outcome criteria you established during the planning step
- determine the extent of outcome achievement—whether the outcome was fully met, partially met, or not met at all
- write evaluation statements
- revise the care plan as needed.

Although technically the last step of the nursing process, evaluation is an ongoing process that occurs each time you see the patient. You must continually evaluate the patient's response to interventions. (See *The focus factor*, below).

A change of plans

If desired outcomes have been achieved, the care plan may be discontinued. If an outcome has been partially met, the plan may be continued with an extended time line.

If a desired outcome hasn't been met, you must reexamine the care plan and make necessary changes. To change the plan, you may need to review the new assessment data, formulate new diagnoses, establish new outcomes, and select new interventions. Then update the written care plan accordingly.

Teacher knows best

Be pliable about care plans

The nursing care plan isn't set in stone. It must be updated as your patient's problems, needs, and priorities change. Be sure to review the care plan often and modify it when necessary.

Teacher knows best

The focus factor

Stay focused during all interactions with your patient. To do this, you'll need to use active listening skills and turn off other unrelated thoughts going through your head. Most patients are aware of the amount of focus and interest you bring to an exchange and will respond in kind.

How the nursing process promotes critical thinking

To use the nursing process, you must be able to think critically. Critical thinking is a disciplined mental process of analyzing problems or phenomena that have been gathered from observation, experience, reflection, reasoning, or communication. Critical thinking while providing patient care, promotes clinical reasoning, which leads to effective decision making.

Deliberate, purposeful, and conscious critical thinking requires reasonable, rational interpretation and evaluation of information. It leads you to reasonable solutions to a problem and helps you choose among these possible solutions to make a decision.

Hallmarks of critical thinking

The hallmarks of critical thinking are:
- clear, careful, and precise thinking
- objective analysis of the evidence
- use of logical reasoning to reach a clinical decision
- elimination of stereotypical thinking, bias, preconceptions, and emotionally charged thinking.

A model process

The nursing process is a model of critical thinking because each step is purposeful, deliberate, and designed to attain a certain goal. (See *Critical thinking: An essential skill.*)

For instance, when evaluating the assessment data you've gathered, you must think critically to determine which questions to ask your patient next. If he says he occasionally experiences chest pain, the critically thinking nurse doesn't simply record this statement and move on to the next topic. Instead, she asks questions designed to elicit details about the chest pain, such as the following:
- When does the pain occur? Do you experience it after strenuous physical activity? Does it occur after meals? While resting?
- How severe is the pain on a scale of 0 to 10?
- Do you have other problems along with the pain?
- Does the pain radiate to other parts of your body?

Risky factors

Thinking critically during assessment enables you to promote safe, quality care by recognizing factors that place your patient at increased risk for developing a problem. If you detect such a potential, you'll know the care plan should include a *Risk for* nursing diagnosis and appropriate interventions to prevent the problem.

Memory jogger

Critical thinking is a life skill as well as a nursing essential. To remember the characteristics of critical-type thought, think of

CLOUD:

Clear

Logical

Objective

Unbiased

Dispassionate (not emotion-driven).

Critical thinking: An essential skill

In the complex, rapidly changing health care environment, safe and effective nursing care demands critical thinking. Taking basic problem solving one step further, critical thinking considers all related factors, including the patient's unique needs and individual differences. Critical-thinking skills allow the nurse to step outside the situation and look at the whole picture more objectively.

Truth seekers

To obtain this complete picture, critical thinkers seek the truth and actively pursue answers to questions. They're also open-minded and creative and can draw from past clinical experience to come up with all possible alternatives and then zero in on the best solution for the patient.

Practice for your practice

Books, articles, and online courses are available to hone nurses' critical-thinking skills. When nurses engage in critical thinking, their patients have the best chances for success.

Likewise, critical thinking helps you write outcomes in a way that promotes easier evaluation and makes the need for any revisions readily apparent.

Novices need it, too

Critical thinking skills are essential for nurses at every level. As a novice nurse, you'll encounter situations you didn't see or learn about during your student clinical rotation—complex problems that require sound decision-making skills. You'll be expected to make important patient care decisions and take actions based on those decisions.

As technology grows more advanced, such decisions and actions are becoming increasingly complex. What's more, they require you to analyze many patient variables, including social, cultural, emotional, physical, financial, and spiritual issues.

Using the nursing process after graduation

No matter how thoroughly you're oriented in your first nursing job, you'll confront many new and unfamiliar situations throughout your career. You'll need to make many on-the-spot decisions—some of which will be crucial. Using the nursing process and critical thinking skills will help you succeed no matter what your responsibilities are. As you become more familiar with the nursing process, gain experience writing care plans, and hone your critical-thinking skills, your clinical judgment and ability to make good decisions undoubtedly will improve.

Roll with the changes

Because the patient's status is dynamic and can change quickly, the nursing process is dynamic as well. As your patient's condition changes, you must assess these changes quickly and adjust the care plan appropriately. Use the nursing process as a road map and critical thinking as the vehicle to take you and your patient to the destination—the desired patient outcome.

Rinse and repeat

As you gain experience, you'll see that the nursing process shows you when and how to stop a nursing intervention—namely, when the desired outcomes are met. Or, if the outcomes remain unmet, the nursing process will lead you to reassess the situation and, if necessary, repeat the entire process.

Understanding NANDA–I, NOC, and NIC

Using standard terminology in the care plan helps ensure that all members of the nursing team have the same understanding of the patient's needs. Technology and the increasing use of electronic medical records have increased the need for standardized nursing language.

Speaking the same language

Several standardized classification systems exist for nursing diagnoses, outcomes, and interventions. With these systems, you can use a single term to describe what otherwise would require several words.

NANDA-I diagnoses

Most nurses use the diagnoses identified by NANDA International (NANDA-I; formerly the North American Nursing Diagnosis Association). NANDA-I develops standardized nursing diagnosis terminology for nurses at all levels and in all practice areas.

NANDA-I was founded in 1973 during a conference held to establish a classification system for nursing diagnoses. In 1987, the American Nurses Association authorized NANDA-I as the governing organization for development of a nursing diagnosis classification system. NANDA-I meets periodically to review and accept new diagnoses or, when necessary, to revise previously accepted diagnoses. It then publishes the updated, revised list of approved diagnoses.

Other classification systems

The Nursing Outcomes Classification (NOC) system, developed at the University of Iowa School of Nursing, is a standardized classification system for patient outcomes that helps nurses evaluate the effects of nursing interventions.

NOC is no laughing matter

NOC outcomes can be used in all settings across the care continuum to follow patient outcomes throughout an illness episode or over an extended time. The NOC system consists of 490 outcomes organized into 32 classes and 7 domains. Each outcome has a definition and a list of measurable indicators. (See *Don't knock NOC!*)

NIC follows NOC

The Nursing Interventions Classification (NIC) system is a comprehensive, research-based standardized classification system for interventions that nurses perform. Like the NOC system, it was developed at the University of Iowa School of Nursing. NIC addresses both the physiological and psychosocial aspects of nursing care and includes independent and collaborative interventions. The NIC system includes 554 interventions organized into 30 classes and 7 domains.

Research conducted and used in formulating NIC helps ensure that nursing interventions are based on the best evidence—not guesswork. Evidence-based interventions promote the best patient outcomes and take the guesswork out of planning care. (See *NIC and nurses*, page 16.)

Weighing the evidence

Don't knock NOC!

Classification of nursing outcomes was initiated in the 1970s in response to a need to identify and measure outcomes of patient care that were responsive to nursing practices. To establish appropriate reimbursement and determine reasonable staffing coverage, health care organizations, insurers, and regulators wanted to measure how the nursing care provided affected the patient's health status. Nurses themselves wanted a language that demonstrated the uniqueness of their profession and provided a framework for further nursing research.

The nursing outcomes listed by the Center for Nursing Classification and Clinical Effectiveness are research based and have been evaluated for reliability, validity, and sensitivity. Therefore, NOC outcomes provide an excellent guideline in the preparation of standardized or individualized care plans, paving the way for evidence-based nursing practice.

Weighing the evidence

NIC and nurses

Research for a classification of nursing interventions began in 1987. Nurses needed a clear, concise, and measurable list of nursing actions to ease documentation time, aid interprofessional communication, assess productivity and competency, foster nursing research, and teach nursing students. These nursing actions were grouped together into broader categories of interventions specific to particular patient outcomes.

For example, the *intervention* "Cardiac Care" contains a list of specific *nursing activities* that partially includes evaluation of chest pain, assessment of peripheral circulation, documentation of cardiac arrhythmia, and promotion of stress reduction. The specific nursing activities listed are based on research and standards of care from relevant professional organizations, and each intervention includes a definition and selected references.

The interventions listed on an individual care plan are ultimately based on the clinical judgment of the nurse responsible for the patient's care. Nursing activities cited must be modified to reflect unique actions required to help that patient meet his/her desired outcomes. Actions that don't apply to the patient should be omitted. This feature of NIC is what guarantees that nurses remain patient focused and in control of the nursing process.

Language linkups

Over the past several years, members of the research teams responsible for NANDA, NIC, and NOC have consulted to develop linkages (terminology that links one classification system to the others). Together, the three classifications provide the basics for a complete care plan. This gives all nurses a common understanding of nursing care.

Concept mapping

A common tool to assist you in critical thinking is a concept map (sometimes called a *mind map*). A concept map is a diagram that shows relationships among various concepts. Concept mapping is a tool for visualizing how concepts relate to one another. It helps you understand your patient's problems and care needs—and see how these items interact with each other.

A concept map helps you organize your thinking and see the big clinical picture. Each concept is enclosed in a box or circle, with lines between related concepts. Concept maps are especially helpful if you're a visual learner.

Comparing concept mapping and care planning

Concept mapping and traditional nursing care planning both have a problem-solving focus. However, concept mapping doesn't require linear design, which can hinder the free flow of ideas. It lets you view information in different ways and from different viewpoints because concepts aren't locked into specific positions. (See *Quick comparison*, below.)

Advantages of concept mapping

Concept mapping also has these other advantages over the traditional care plan:
- It makes the seemingly intangible concepts of patient problems, causes, and effects more manageable.
- It clearly defines the central concept (the patient problem) by positioning it in the center of the page. This ensures that the patient—not the medical diagnosis—is the focus.

Quick comparison

Here's a quick comparison of concept mapping and nursing care plans.

Concept map	Nursing care plan
• Visually organized	• Linearly organized
• Assessment data usually in separate area or different form	• Assessment data clearly linked to nursing problems (diagnoses)
• Good for quick communication of priority problems, outcomes, and interventions	• Good for quick identification and outline of multiple patient problems

- It shows the relative importance of each concept.
- It helps you identify connections between important concepts.
- It requires much less time to write than does a care plan.
- It encourages creative and innovative ideas.
- It provides all the basic information on one page.
- It allows new information to be easily added.
- It enables you to see contradictions and gaps in the material or its interpretation, which provides a foundation for questioning, discovery, and creativity.

Concept mapping is similar to the brain's neural network. Each concept has long fibers that reach out and connect to other concepts.

Disadvantages of concept mapping

Despite its advantages, concept mapping can have certain drawbacks:

- Getting the map just right can be time-consuming. You may have to redraw it several times until you're satisfied.
- It may become complex and cluttered, hindering your ability to see the big picture.
- It doesn't easily lend itself to standardized formats for everyday use in the clinical setting.

Creating a concept map

B.R.
Chief complaint
- RLQ pain
- Nausea, vomiting
- Fever
Medical diagnosis
Appendicitis

To develop a concept map for your patient, start with a clean sheet of unlined paper. (If you must use lined paper, turn it so the lines are vertical.) To promote creative thinking, you may want to use colored pencils or pens. Then follow these steps:

- After you've assessed your patient, place a circle representing the patient in the middle of the paper. In this circle, write the patient's name or initials, chief complaint, and medical diagnosis. (See example at left.) By placing the patient in the center of the page, your focus is clearly patient centered. Remember, be brief!
- Write the patient's major problems or nursing diagnoses in boxes surrounding the patient, along with pertinent supporting data.
- Use lines to connect the central circle—the patient—to the nursing diagnoses boxes. You may also draw lines between related nursing diagnoses. For example, for a postoperative patient experiencing constipation caused by use of opioid analgesics, you would draw a line between the nursing diagnoses of *Acute pain* and *Constipation* to show that you understand they're related. (See example at right.)
- Write expected outcomes for each nursing diagnosis; place each outcome in its own box because corresponding interventions will

Acute pain
- Verbalized incisional pain
- Rates pain as 9 on pain scale

B.R.
Chief complaint
- RLQ pain
- Nausea, vomiting
- Fever
Medical diagnosis
Appendicitis

Constipation
- Distended abdomen
- Inability to pass stool

Concept mapping without tears

These guidelines can help you to learn how to quickly and easily create concept maps:
• Work quickly without pausing. Try to keep up with the flow of ideas. Don't stop to decide where something should go or to organize the material. Just get it down on paper. Ordering and analyzing are linear activities that can disrupt the mapping process.
• Write down everything you can think of without judging or editing—these activities can also disrupt the flow of concept mapping.
• If you come to a standstill, look over what you've done to see if you've left anything out.
• Confine the map to one page so it's easier to use.
• Print in capital letters for greater legibility. This also encourages you to keep the points brief.
• Initially, you may want to use color coding to group sections of the map. As you gain experience, you'll probably find that color coding isn't necessary.

differ for each outcome. Connect these boxes with lines to the appropriate nursing diagnosis.
• In the same way, write interventions in a box for each outcome, followed by evaluations. Draw lines between each part of the nursing process to link related concepts. (See *Concept mapping without tears*.)

Patterns, symbols, and notes

To help clarify your concept map, try using patterns and symbols to help organize types of information, such as:
• branches, to show how a concept can branch into ideas that are either closely or distantly related
• arrows, to join ideas from different branches
• circled groupings, to combine several branches of related ideas.
You may also include explanatory notes—such as a few words, phrases, or sentences—to explain, question, or comment on a particular point.

Using your concept map

Concept maps are such useful tools that they can be used for multiple purposes. For example, you can use a concept map to analyze a case study for class or to guide your patient care during clinical rotations. During clinical practicum, you can carry your concept map in your pocket or place it on your clipboard so you can refer to it often and update or revise it as necessary.

On the case

Case study background

Mr. Jones is a 58-year-old male who was admitted to the medical-surgical floor with cholecystitis. The patient complains of pain in his epigastric area, nausea, and vomiting. His vital signs are as follows: heart rate 102 beats/minute, blood pressure 142/88 mm Hg, oral temperature 100.4°F, and respiratory rate 22 breaths/minute.

The patient rates his pain as an 8 on a scale of 0 to 10, with 10 being the most severe pain possible and 0 being the absence of pain. A nasogastric (NG) tube has been placed and is connected to low, intermittent wall suction, and an IV line with dextrose 5% in normal saline solution has been started at 75 mL/hour. Mr. Jones is scheduled for a laparoscopic cholecystectomy tomorrow.

Concept mapping exercise

Follow the steps outlined here to create a rough concept map for the care of Mr. Jones. Don't worry if you can't complete the entire care plan. This is just your first try. The answers can be found on page 21.

Steps

1. Assess the patient to collect clinical data.
2. Write the patient's name or initials, medical diagnosis, and chief complaint in the middle of a sheet of paper.
3. Write appropriate nursing diagnoses in boxes around the central box that contains the patient's name or initials and chief complaint. (*Hint:* One of the diagnoses should be *Acute pain.*)
4. Categorize assessment data under the appropriate nursing diagnoses.
5. Analyze the relationships among nursing diagnoses and draw lines to indicate these relationships.
6. On another piece of paper, identify patient goals, expected outcomes, and nursing interventions for the nursing diagnosis *Acute pain.* Or, instead of using another piece of paper, you can create additional boxes on your concept map for the goals, outcomes, and interventions and then link these boxes to the related nursing diagnoses.

Answer key

Concept mapping exercise

Steps 1, 2, 3, 4, and 5

This concept map is one example of many possibilities for this patient. If you couldn't complete this concept map, don't worry. The remaining chapters in this book will walk you step-by-step through the process of creating a concept map that incorporates each stage of the nursing process.

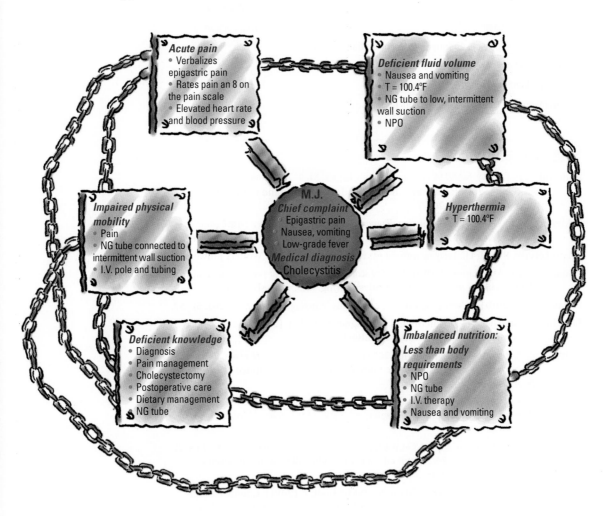

Acute pain
- Verbalizes epigastric pain
- Rates pain an 8 on the pain scale
- Elevated heart rate and blood pressure

Deficient fluid volume
- Nausea and vomiting
- T = 100.4°F
- NG tube to low, intermittent wall suction
- NPO

Impaired physical mobility
- Pain
- NG tube connected to intermittent wall suction
- I.V. pole and tubing

M.J.
Chief complaint
- Epigastric pain
- Nausea, vomiting
- Low-grade fever
Medical diagnosis
Cholecystitis

Hyperthermia
- T = 100.4°F

Deficient knowledge
- Diagnosis
- Pain management
- Cholecystectomy
- Postoperative care
- Dietary management
- NG tube

Imbalanced nutrition: Less than body requirements
- NPO
- NG tube
- I.V. therapy
- Nausea and vomiting

Step 6

Here's an example of a goal, expected outcomes, and nursing interventions for the nursing diagnosis *Acute pain*:

- *Nursing diagnosis:* Acute pain related to inflammation of the gallbladder as evidenced by the patient reporting pain rating as an 8 on a 0-to-10 scale
  - ○ *Nursing priority:* Pain control
- *Expected outcome:* Patient's self-reported pain level is reduced to 3 on a 0-to-10 scale within 2 hours of initiation of prescribed analgesics.

Nursing interventions	Evaluation
Assess pain using pain scale.	*This section will include the patient's responses to the interventions on the left.*
Medicate patient for pain, according to the practitioner's orders.	
Instruct patient on use of patient-controlled analgesia, if appropriate.	
Position patient for comfort.	
Use techniques of relaxation, meditation, or guided imagery.	

Selected references

Abdejalil, E. R. (2016). *NANDA nursing diagnosis list for 2015–2017*. Retrieved on November 2016 from: http://health-conditions.com/nanda-nursing-diagnosis-list-2015-2017/

Ackley, B., & Ladwig, G. (2014) *Nursing diagnosis handbook: An evidence-based guide to planning care* (10th ed.). Maryland Heights, St Louis, MO: Mosby Elsevier.

Alfaro-LeFevre, R. (2014). *Applying nursing process*. Philadelphia, PA: Wolters Kluwer.

American Nurse Association. (2015). *Nursing scope and standards of performance and standards of clinical practice* (3rd ed.). Silver Spring, MD: nursesbooks.org.

Ballantyne, H. (2016). Developing nursing care plans. *Nursing Standard, 30*(26), 51–57.

Bulechek, G., Butcher, H., Dochterman, J., & Wagner, C. (Eds.). (2013). *Nursing interventions class (NIC)*. St. Louis, MO: Elsevier.

Continuing Professional Development. (2015). *Developing nursing care plans*. Retrieved on November 2016 from: http://journals.rcni.com/doi/pdfplus/10.7748/ns.30.26.51.s48

Cronenwett, L., Sherwood, G., Barnsteiner, J., Disch, J., Johnson, J., Mitchell, P., ... Warren, J. (2007). Quality and safety education for nurses. *Nursing Outlook, 55*(3), 122–131.

Herdman, H., & Kamitsuru, S. *NANDA international, Inc. nursing diagnoses: Definitions & classification, 2015–2017* (10th ed.). Oxford: Wiley Blackwell. Retrieved on November 2016 from: http://iaud.ac.ir

Moattari, M., Soleimani, S., Moghaddam, N., & Mehbodi, F. (2014). *Clinical concept mapping: Does it improve discipline-based critical thinking of nursing students?*. Retrieved on November 2016 from: https://www.ncbi.nlm.nih.gov/pmc/articles/PMC3917188/

Moorehead, S., Johnson, M., Maas, M., & Swanson, E. (Eds.). (2013). *Nursing outcomes classification (NOC)* (5th ed.). St. Louis, MO: Elsevier.

Papathanasiou, I., Kleisiaris, C., Fradelos, E., Kakou, K., & Kourkouta, L. (2014). *Critical thinking: The development of an essential skill for nursing students.* Retrieved on November 2016 from: https://www.ncbi.nlm.nih.gov/pmc/articles/PMC4216424/

Price, B. (2015). *Applying critical thinking to nursing.* Retrieved on November 2016 from: http://journals.rcni.com/doi/pdfplus/10.7748/ns.29.51.49.e10005

QSEN Competencies. Retrieved on January 23, 2017 from: http://qsen.org/competencies/pre-licensure-ksas/

Ralph, S., & Taylor, C. (2014). *Nursing diagnosis reference manual.* Philadelphia, PA: Wolters Kluwer.

Shoulders, B., Follet, C., & Eason, J. (2014). *Enhancing critical thinking in clinical practice: Implications for critical and acute care nurses.* Retrieved on November 2016 from: http://journals.lww.com/dccnjournal/Fulltext/2014/07000/Enhancing_Critical_Thinking_in_Clinical_Practice_.5.aspx

University of Iowa, College of Nursing. (2013). *CNC—overview: Nursing outcomes classification (NOC).* Retrieved on November 2016 from: https://nursing.uiowa.edu/cncce/nursing-outcomes-classification-overview

University of Iowa, College of Nursing. (2013). *CNC—overview: Nursing interventions classification (NIC).* Retrieved on November 2016 from: https://nursing.uiowa.edu/cncce/nursing-interventions-classification-overview

Chapter 2

Assessment

Just the facts

In this chapter, you'll learn:

◆ the components of a complete health assessment

◆ techniques and formats for gathering and organizing assessment data

◆ tips for reviewing a patient's chart for assessment data

◆ the steps for creating a concept map using assessment information.

A look at assessment

The first step in the nursing process, assessment, involves data collection to identify the patient's actual and potential health problems and needs. The goal is to gather as much information about your patient as possible. Using these data, you'll identify his needs, formulate nursing diagnoses, establish expected outcomes, and identify interventions to help achieve those expected outcomes. You'll also set objective criteria to evaluate the effectiveness of your interventions.

Can I read that back to you?

Be sure to double-check, clarify, or restate the information you've collected to make sure that it's accurate and complete. Validating the data helps you avoid misinterpretation. Remember, if your assessment is incorrect or incomplete, the nursing diagnoses you formulate are likely to be incorrect as well or you may overlook a problem and neglect to formulate a diagnosis for it.

Also, to make sure that the data you've gathered accurately reflect the patient's life experiences and living patterns, maintain an objective, nonjudgmental approach during assessment.

Think of the nursing assessment as a fact-finding mission.

Complete vs. focused assessment

Depending on the situation and time constraints, your assessment may be complete or focused.

You complete me

A *complete* assessment provides comprehensive baseline information. Typically, it's conducted when the patient is admitted. Student nurses are generally expected to perform a complete assessment as part of their learning experience.

Hocus focus

A *focused* assessment generally is problem or need oriented. During this assessment, focus on evaluating for specific problems or concerns that have already been identified and are being tracked by the health care team until they're resolved.

Typically, you'll perform a focused assessment after the patient has been admitted and undergone a complete assessment—for example, during initial shift assessment or change of assignment, whenever the patient has a new complaint or a change in condition, or when you're evaluating the results of an intervention.

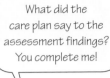

What did the care plan say to the assessment findings? You complete me!

Components of a complete health assessment

A complete health assessment includes the:
- nursing history
- physical assessment
- review of laboratory and diagnostic test results
- review of other available health information.

First impressions

Assessment begins as soon as you meet your patient. Perhaps without even being aware of it, you're already noting such aspects as his skin color, speech patterns, and body position. Your education as a nurse gives you the ability to organize and interpret these data. As you move on to conduct the formal nursing assessment, you'll collect data in a more structured way. The findings you collect from your assessment may be subjective or objective. (See *Subjective vs. objective findings*.)

Group dynamics

When evaluating the assessment data, you'll start to recognize significant points and ask pertinent questions. You'll probably find yourself starting to group related bits of significant assessment data into clusters that give you clues about your patient's problem and prompt additional questions. For instance, if the data suggest a pattern of poor nutrition, you should ask questions that will help elicit the cause, such as the following:
- Do you have a poor appetite?
- Do you eat most meals alone?
- Do you have enough money to buy food?

Subjective vs. objective findings

Keep in mind that assessment findings fall into two broad categories: subjective and objective.

Subjective data

Subjective assessment data represent the perception or reality experienced by the person reporting the information. It may come directly from the patient or indirectly from family members, caregivers, or other health care providers. For example, when you ask a patient to rate his pain on a scale of 0 to 10, you're asking him to quantify his personal perception of the severity of his pain. Even indirect data can provide clues that could prove vital to your patient's care. In some cases—for instance, if your patient is physically or mentally incapable of answering questions or providing information—such third-party sources are crucial to your assessment.

Objective data

Objective data come from the physical examination through inspection, percussion, palpation, and auscultation. Use physical findings to verify the subjective findings you've gathered from the patient's health history. For example, diminished breath sounds heard on auscultation of the lower lobes of the lungs (objective data) support the patient's report of "having trouble breathing" (subjective data).

On the other hand, if the patient reports frequent nausea, you should suspect that this may be the cause of his poor nutrition. Therefore, you'd ask questions to elicit more information about this symptom, such as the following:
- Do you feel nauseated after meals? Before meals?
- Do any of your medications upset your stomach?

History

The nursing history requires you to collect information about the patient's:
- biographic data
- current physical and emotional concerns or problems
- current medications, prescription or over-the-counter or herbal supplements, and allergies to medications or other substances
- past medical and surgical history
- past and current ability to perform activities of daily living (ADLs)
- availability of support systems, effectiveness of past coping patterns, and perceived stressors
- socioeconomic factors affecting preventive health practices and compliance with medical recommendations
- spiritual and cultural practices, wishes, or concerns

- sexuality, gender identity, sexual practices, plans for pregnancy, and use of contraceptives
- family patterns of illness and any history of genetic disorders in the family.

Biographic data

Begin your history by obtaining biographic data from the patient. Do this before you begin gathering details about his health. Ask the patient his name, address, telephone number, birth date, age, marital status, religion, and nationality. Find out who the patient lives with and get the name and number of a person to contact in case of an emergency. Also ask the patient about his health care, including the name of his primary practitioner and his mode of transportation to practitioner visits. Finally, ask the patient if he has an advance directive and, if not, if he wants more information on advance directives.

If the patient can't furnish accurate information, ask him for the name of a friend or relative who can. However, be aware that gathering information from a person other than the patient may be biased or inaccurate. Always document the source of the information you collect as well as whether an interpreter was necessary. It is a responsibility of the health care institution to provide an interpreter for patients who do not speak English. The patient is the BEST source of information about their health. The nurse should also assess the reliability of the patient as a historian and note this.

Current complaints

To explore the patient's current complaints, ask the patient why he's seeking health care. Patient complaints provide valuable data immediately. When you explore these initial complaints, you may uncover crucial additional information.

Digging in the dirt

Record the patient's current health concerns or problems in his own words. Ask him to describe the problem in detail, including any suspected cause. Ask about the onset and location of the symptoms, characteristics of the symptoms, duration, time, and setting in which the symptoms occur. Ask the patient what relieves the symptoms or what factors aggravate the symptoms. If the patient has pain, ask him to evaluate it on a scale of 0 to 10, 10 being the worst pain he has ever experienced.

Also ask the patient if he is taking any medications, including over-the-counter (OTC) preparations, such as aspirin, vitamins, or supplements. If so, how much do you take and how often do you take it? Do you use home remedies such as homemade ointments? Do you use herbal preparations or take dietary supplements? Do you use other alternative or complementary therapies, such as acupuncture, massage, or chiropractic?

Also ask the patient if he is allergic to anything in the environment or to any drugs or foods. If so, what kind of allergic reaction do you have?

Recording your patient's complaints in his own words is good nursing practice.

Past medical history

Ask the patient about past medical problems and surgical procedures. Typical questions include the following:

- Have you ever been hospitalized? If so, when and why?
- Did you have any childhood illnesses? Up to date on immunizations?
- Are you currently being treated for any problem, such as hypertension or diabetes? If so, for what problem and who is your practitioner?
- Have you ever had surgery? If so, when and why?

Family history

- What illnesses are in the family? Does the patient know of any genetic disorders in the family?
- If there is a genetic disorder in the family, you can draw a genogram to illustrate this (*see illustration of genogram*).

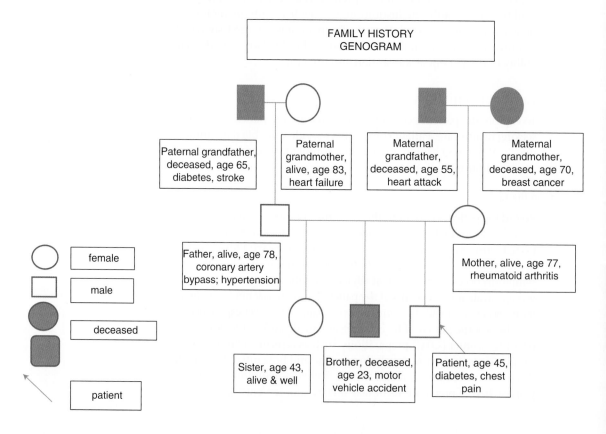

FAMILY HISTORY GENOGRAM

Paternal grandfather, deceased, age 65, diabetes, stroke

Paternal grandmother, alive, age 83, heart failure

Maternal grandfather, deceased, age 55, heart attack

Maternal grandmother, deceased, age 70, breast cancer

Father, alive, age 78, coronary artery bypass; hypertension

Mother, alive, age 77, rheumatoid arthritis

Sister, age 43, alive & well

Brother, deceased, age 23, motor vehicle accident

Patient, age 45, diabetes, chest pain

female

male

deceased

patient

- Are the patient's parents alive? Do they have any disorders? What are their ages? If deceased, what were their health problems and age of death?
- Is anyone in the family currently ill? What problem or disorder is occurring?

Activities of daily living (ADLs)

Find out about your patient's ability to perform ADLs by asking him to describe his typical day. The types of information you seek should include:
- appetite, special diets, food allergies, and meal preparation
- urinary and bowel elimination habits
- exercise and sleep habits and any aids required for sleep
- work and leisure activities and recent travel
- use of tobacco, alcohol, marijuana, and other drugs
- religious or spiritual needs of the patient
- sexually transmitted diseases, sexual practices, and partners
- plans of pregnancy and contraceptives used.
  Also, be sure to elicit the patient's view of how the present illness has affected his usual performance of ADLs.

Support systems and stressors

Because illness doesn't occur in isolation, you also need to ask about other aspects of your patient's life, including the availability of support systems and perceived stressors, when you collect your history data. These other life factors can enhance or complicate a patient's condition or affect his recovery.

Thank you for being a friend

For instance, lack of social support can affect a patient's physical well-being and influence patient outcomes. In addition to family members, a patient's social support system may include partners, friends, coworkers, community agencies, vocational groups, and clergy who provide assistance in times of anxiety or crisis.

You can begin your evaluation of your patient's support system by asking the patient, "Who's with you today?" or "How did you get here today?" Other questions that elicit information about the patient's support system include the following:
- Do you live alone? Do you need to climb stairs in your home?
- Is anyone available to assist you at home, if needed?
- Who provides emotional support for you and is this adequate?
- More intimate details of the patient's social support system are usually best obtained in ongoing interactions during caregiving activities or as you and the patient begin to discuss discharge plans. As appropriate, weave the information you obtain about your patient's support system into the care plan.

Stress marks

Emotional, social, and physical demands on the body cause stress. The amount of stress a patient experiences can affect his physiological and psychological health. To elicit information about your patient's stress level and methods of coping with stress, ask:

- what situations he finds stressful
- how he responds physically to stress
- what he does when he feels stress
- whether stress affects his family relationships
- if he thinks stress affects his health.

Also, inquire about potential stressors, such as recent losses or setbacks, spiritual concerns, difficulties with self-care or normal ADLs, and exposure to abuse (see *Asking about abuse*). These may be important clues that help you formulate a care plan.

Socioeconomic factors

The patient's socioeconomic status can directly affect health behaviors by determining the financial resources available for health care and a healthful lifestyle, including adequate housing, clothing, and nutrition. For example, a patient whose insurance plan doesn't reimburse routine health screening and physical examinations usually seeks health care only for illness. Similarly, a patient whose financial resources barely meet basic needs is less likely to use services or products designed to promote or maintain health.

Asking about abuse

A history of abuse is an important aspect of a patient's psychosocial history. Remember that anyone can be a victim of abuse, including a boyfriend or girlfriend, a spouse, an elderly person, a child, or a parent. In addition, abuse can occur in many forms, including physical, psychological, emotional, and sexual abuse.

When taking a health history, you should ask two questions to explore abuse:

- When do you feel safe at home?
- When do you not feel safe at home?

Reaction time

Even when you don't immediately suspect an abusive situation, be aware of how your patient reacts to open-ended questions. Is the patient defensive, hostile, confused, or frightened? Assess how the patient interacts with you and others. Does he seem withdrawn or frightened or show other inappropriate behavior? Keep his reactions in mind when you perform your physical assessment.

Remember to report

Remember, if the patient tells you about any type of abuse, you're obligated to report it. Inform the patient that you must report the incident to local authorities.

Insurance plan

To assess health-related socioeconomic factors, find out if your patient has health insurance and, if so, whether insurance pays for a routine physical examination or other screening procedures. Also find out whether the patient is receiving financial aid and whether his income is sufficient to pay for housing, food, and clothing.

Spiritual and cultural influences

Some patients attach great importance to their spiritual and religious beliefs. Spirituality (one's personal definition of the purpose and meaning of life and the world) may assign meaning to individual and community life, guide daily behavior and lifestyle, define acceptable health care, and influence attitudes toward illness and death.

Divine thing

Religion is the component of spirituality that includes particular practices related to a belief in a divine power. A religious system usually embraces more specific beliefs, including prescribed behaviors, rituals, or practices. A patient's health beliefs and practices may be linked closely to religion.

Culture club

A patient's cultural background can also profoundly influence his views of life and death, health beliefs, health and dietary habits, roles, relationships, and family dynamics. For example, patients from some cultures avoid seeking health care or taking responsibility for changing unhealthful behaviors because they feel powerless to control their illness, which they may consider punishment for some wrongdoing. To find out about your patient's spiritual and cultural influences, ask these questions:
• Do you have religious or cultural beliefs that affect your diet or health practices?
• Would you like me to contact any religious affiliation for you?
Assessing cultural influences can bring health-related factors to light and identify culturally related strengths, such as a strong support system.

Lost in translation?

If the patient has a language barrier, talk with your manager or the family to assist you in finding an interpreter. When you first interact with the patient with an interpreter present, explain the facility's basic routines and establish a functional method of communicating about important health issues, such as pain, constipation, nausea, or other common symptoms. This is also a good time to verify that the patient understands use of the call light and any treatments or restrictions ordered.

When assessing your patient's spiritual beliefs, don't let your own beliefs color your attitude. Remember to remain nonjudgmental.

All in the family history

Being aware of patterns of illness in families can help you understand genetic risk factors, determine the influence of these events on the attitudes of your patient, and plan effective interventions. For example, a 49-year-old male with a family history of several male deaths from heart attack before age 50 who experiences chest pain may be significantly more afraid or hopeless than a peer with a similar complaint but no early male cardiac deaths in his family.

In some clinical settings, you may not have access to a family medical history because it's obtained by the practitioner but isn't immediately available to you. In this case, obtain a brief history of relevant illness in the patient's parents, siblings, and, when indicated, grandparents. Typical questions include the following:

• Are your mother, father, and siblings living?
• If not, how old were they when they died? What were the causes of their deaths?
• If they're alive, do they have diabetes, high blood pressure, heart disease, asthma, cancer, sickle cell anemia, hemophilia, cataracts, glaucoma, or other illnesses?

Show a little respect

Being observant, open, and interested are commonly the best ways to learn about other people's spiritual and cultural viewpoints. Whether you're asking questions or responding to patient queries, be careful to avoid making assumptions about people who might be ethnically or culturally different from you. A simple question opener such as "Would you be comfortable if I...?" can demonstrate your respect for the patient's feelings and your willingness to adapt your care to the patient's needs.

Physical examination

During the physical examination, you obtain data using four of your five senses—sight, hearing, touch, and smell. A complete examination includes a general survey, measurement of vital signs, height and weight measurements, and assessment of all organs and body systems. (See *Examining the goals of a physical examination*.) This type of examination is appropriate for periodic health checks. Of course, in many cases, you won't have time for a complete examination and will need to focus on particular complaints or health problems.

General survey

The general survey provides vital information about the patient's behavior and health status. During your first contact with the patient, expect to receive a steady stream of impressions—most of which are visual. The patient's gender, race, and approximate age will generally be obvious. Because some health concerns may relate to these factors, be sure to note them.

Examining the goals of a physical examination

During the physical examination, keep in mind that your goal as a nurse is to identify signs, symptoms, and problems for which the patient needs nursing interventions. In other words, the data you collect should lead you to formulate a nursing diagnosis—not a medical diagnosis. The nurse's focus is always on patient processes.

Medical practitioners (such as doctors, nurse practitioners, and physician assistants), on the other hand, use a method called *differential diagnosis* to arrive at a medical diagnosis. After identifying signs and symptoms, they systematically eliminate related diagnoses until they identify and substantiate a precise diagnosis by objective means, such as radiologic or laboratory findings. The practitioner's focus is the disease processes.

Meaningful collaboration among practitioners and nurses leads to health care that maximizes the patient's health and quality of life or preserves his comfort and dignity in death.

Also note less-obvious factors that can contribute to an overall impression, including:

- signs of distress
- orientation to time, place, and person
- facial characteristics
- body type, posture, and movements
- speech
- dress
- grooming and personal hygiene
- style of interacting with others.

Summarize

When you've completed the survey, document your initial impressions of the patient in a one-paragraph statement—a summary that gives an overall picture to guide your subsequent examination.

Physical examination techniques

To perform the physical examination, you'll use four basic techniques—inspection, palpation, percussion, and auscultation.

All eyes on inspection

Inspection, or critical observation, is the most frequently used assessment technique. Performed correctly, it also reveals more than the other techniques. But incomplete or hasty inspection may neglect important details or yield false or misleading findings.

To ensure accurate, useful information, approach inspection in a careful, unhurried manner. Pay close attention to details as you assess each body system, observing for color, size, location, movement, texture, symmetry, odors, and sounds. Try to draw logical conclusions from the findings.

Palpation points

Inform the patient that you need to palpate different areas to examine them. During palpation, you touch the patient's body with your hands, using various degrees of pressure to feel pulsations and vibrations, locate body structures, and assess such characteristics as size, texture, warmth, mobility, and tenderness. Palpation allows you to detect a pulse, muscle rigidity, enlarged lymph nodes, skin dryness, organ tenderness, or breast lumps as well as measure chest expansion and contraction during respiration.

Percussion discussion

During percussion, you tap your fingers or hands quickly and sharply against body surfaces (usually the chest and abdomen) to produce sounds, detect tenderness, or assess reflexes. Percussion for sound (the most common goal) helps locate organ borders, identify organ shape and position, and determine if an organ is solid or filled with fluid or gas.

Listen closely

Auscultation involves listening to body sounds—especially those produced by the heart, lungs, blood vessels, stomach, and intestines. For all but the most pronounced body sounds, you'll need a stethoscope to auscultate.

Don't forget that inspection is an important part of the physical exam.

Diagnostic testing data

Make sure that you know how to access the patient's laboratory and other diagnostic test results. In most record-keeping systems, laboratory results are printed or electronically formatted on forms that specify what laboratory performed the test, the normal range of values for that test, the patient's test value, and where that value lies in relation to the normal range. Remember that "normal" values for many tests vary somewhat between different laboratories, depending on the specific equipment or testing techniques they use. In a student nursing care plan, always cite the normal range listed for the laboratory performing the test.

Other test results may be filed by type or located by date of service. Radiology, nuclear scanning, computed tomography, magnetic resonance imaging, and ultrasound results commonly are kept together. Endoscopic and biopsy reports may be filed separately, with the report containing a section on the procedure process as well as the specific findings. Electrocardiograms are commonly kept together for ease of comparison.

Supporting role

Nurses not only need to be aware of what tests the patient has had and the results but should have an understanding of the disease process and what these results may mean. Patients may be understandably anxious about the details of preparing for or going through a particular test, how soon results will be available, and what these results mean. The nurse is responsible for teaching and preparing the patient and then identifying and responding to posttest complications or reactions. The practitioner is responsible for conveying test results and implications to the patient, but nurses are commonly asked to review and clarify the information provided as the patient thinks through what he has been told.

Other health information in the patient's chart

The patient's chart is an excellent source of assessment data. Always review it carefully, including assessments made by other health care team members, such as emergency department (ED) staff, the admitting practitioner, consulting medical specialists, other nursing staff and advanced practice consultants, dietitians, physical or other specialty therapy personnel, pharmacy consultants, social service workers, and discharge planners. The practitioner's history and physical examination findings can guide your questioning during assessment. If appropriate, you should attempt to corroborate these findings during the nursing assessment. If your assessment findings differ, report your findings as appropriate.

Get to know your patient's medication list inside and out. It may affect your care plan. Getting to know you...

Medication use

Be sure to review your patient's current medication use. Ask about prescription drugs, OTC drugs, and herbal remedies. List these medications on the patient's chart when he's admitted to the facility. Medications that are prescribed during hospitalization are listed on a medication administration record (MAR). Look closely at the details of each drug order.

Look before you leap

Before your clinical rotation or first patient contact, check your patient's list of prescribed drugs and their dosages and make sure that you know what adverse reactions and interactions these drugs could cause. Also find out if the patient understands the purpose of each drug; this will help determine if he needs additional teaching during hospitalization or at discharge. If appropriate, ask about the patient's previous medication use as well, find out if he experienced adverse reactions, and ask about recreational drug use.

If you question a drug, dosage, or route listed on the MAR, double-check the original order in the medical record first and then call the pharmacy or practitioner as appropriate. In the home care setting, check the labels on the patient's prescriptions and call the pharmacy or the practitioner to validate discrepancies between the labels, the patient's statements, and the physician orders in the nursing record.

Medical procedure data

Review the medical procedures scheduled for your patient. Knowing which procedures the patient is scheduled for can help you anticipate potential problems and alert you to postprocedure signs and symptoms to watch for.

For example...

If the patient is scheduled for myelography, you would expect to verify the allergy history, looking particularly for an allergy to iodine or other contrast materials, and notify the referring practitioner and radiologist of new information. You would also expect to explain to the patient what's going to happen before, during, and after the procedure, including transfer to the radiology suite, and instruct him about procedure restrictions, including the need to:

- withhold solid foods and certain medications before the test
- void right before the test
- remove any jewelry
- maintain a sidelying, fetal-type position during injection of the contrast medium into the spinal canal by the radiologist just before the test.

Similarly, if the patient has just undergone a procedure involving anesthetics or other medications, you would know to assess for adverse reactions to these agents.

Admitting medical diagnosis

You should also review the patient's medical diagnosis. Determine if your patient's current concerns and assessment findings match his admitting diagnosis. If you uncover new information, report it to the practitioner because these new findings may affect the treatment plan. Make sure you understand the meaning and implications of your patient's medical diagnosis—including its pathophysiology, signs and symptoms, required diagnostic tests, treatments, complications, preparation for procedures, and postprocedure care. This information helps you focus your assessment.

Special consideration

If your patient is diagnosed with ulcerative colitis, for instance, you would realize that he's more prone to develop anemia due to internal bleeding. Consequently, you would be sure to monitor his hematology reports, check his vital signs frequently, and observe elimination patterns and changes. On the other hand, for a patient admitted with diabetes mellitus, you would stay alert for signs and symptoms of hypoglycemia or hyperglycemia.

Data collection and organization

Every nurse must know how to collect and organize patient data in a meaningful format. Doing this helps you formulate correct nursing diagnoses and allows other health care team members to readily understand the data you've documented.

In your educational process, you are often asked to organize your information by functional health patterns. In the clinical setting, many different types of integrated or specialty assessment database formats may be used, according to the regulations and specific requirements for that facility.

Gordon's functional health patterns

To organize and analyze the patient data you collect, you may want to use the functional health patterns and rating scale proposed in 1987 by Marjory Gordon. Gordon's functional health categories include:

- health perception and management
- nutrition and metabolism
- elimination
- activity and exercise
- cognition and perception
- sleep and rest
- self-perception and self-concept
- sexuality and reproduction
- roles and relationships
- coping and stress management
- values and beliefs.

These 11 categories provide a framework for a systematic, standardized approach to data collection.

You can use Gordon's functional health patterns to obtain a nursing history from the patient's perspective through a series of specific questions. These patterns are flexible and adaptable and can be used for patients in various states of health, from different age groups, and in different clinical settings. Gordon's functional health patterns have also become an integral part of many nursing database documentation systems.

The data you collect on your patient can be overwhelming. Good thing that there are systems for organizing all these data.

Assigning functional level codes

Some facilities require nurses to assign codes during patient assessment to describe the patient's functional level according to Gordon's functional health patterns (as shown at right). This type of scale has been adapted to many settings and uses, particularly in long-term care assessments of activities of daily living. As a student, your instructor may also require you to grade the patient's functional level.

Grading system

If you're asked to assign functional level codes, you'll grade the functional level of the patient on a scale of 0 to 4 in each of the 11 categories described in the text. You'll also assign a code that most closely describes the patient's overall functional level.

Code name "Outcomes"

Functional levels can also be incorporated into your expected outcomes. To do this, you would include a reference to the functional level you expect the patient to attain as a result of your nursing interventions and other collaborative care. Say, for example, a patient is receiving rehabilitation after a hip fracture repair. Based on your initial assessment, you rate his functional mobility level as 3 because he requires supervision to stand up and walk safely with a walker. Your expected outcome statement might read: "Attains functional mobility level of 1 as demonstrated by standing up and walking 15′ with a cane, unassisted, by discharge." You'll read more about writing outcome statements in Chapter 4, Planning.

LEVEL 4

LEVEL 3

LEVEL 2

LEVEL 1

LEVEL 0

INDEPENDENT

Deciphering code

To document your patient's functional health patterns, you'll assign a code based on a five-point scale that rates the ability of the patient to function independently. (See *Assigning functional level codes*.) By focusing on each health pattern in turn, you can better evaluate your patient's overall level of health and well-being.

Health perception and management

To obtain data about the health perception and management pattern, ask questions that help determine the patient's:
- perception of his level of health
- detrimental habits, such as smoking or excessive alcohol use
- actual or potential problems related to safety and health management or the need for home modifications or continued care at home.

Activity and exercise

When evaluating the patient's activity and exercise pattern, assess:
- the patient's ability to manage normal ADLs that require energy expenditure, including self-care, exercise, and leisure time
- major body systems involved with activity and exercise (respiratory, cardiovascular, and musculoskeletal systems).

Nutrition and metabolism

To assess nutrition and metabolism, ask the patient questions about:
- food and fluid consumption relative to metabolic needs
- adequacy of nourishment
- dietary habits and preferences
- any dietary restrictions
- problems related to fluid balance, tissue integrity, adequate nutrition, and immunologic defenses
- GI problems.

Gordon says that nutrition and metabolism are one of the 11 functional health categories.

Elimination

To assess your patient's elimination pattern, ask questions related to his excretory patterns (bowel, bladder, and skin) and check for such problems as incontinence, constipation, diarrhea, and urine retention.

Sleep and rest

When assessing the patient's sleep and rest pattern, inquire about:
- sleep, rest, and relaxation practices
- dysfunctional sleep patterns, fatigue, and responses to sleep deprivation.

Cognition and perception

To assess cognition and perception, evaluate the patient's:
- ability to comprehend and use information
- sensory and neurologic functions
- sensory experiences, such as pain and altered sensory input.

Self-perception and self-concept

To assess your patient's self-perception and self-concept, evaluate:
- attitudes toward self, including identity, body image, self-worth, and self-esteem
- response to threats to self-concept.

Sexuality and reproduction

To assess the patient's sexuality and reproduction pattern, evaluate:
- sexuality concerns
- sexual practices
- for female patients, last menstrual period
- any past sexually transmitted disease
- use of safe sex practices
- past pregnancies and types of delivery
- plans for pregnancy
- use of contraceptives or hormones.

Roles and relationships

To assess your patient's roles and relationships, evaluate:
- roles in the world and relationships with others
- role in the family
- satisfaction with roles
- role strain
- dysfunctional relationships.

Coping and stress management

Explore your patient's coping and stress management pattern by asking questions about his:
- perception of stress and coping strategies
- support systems
- symptoms of stress
- effectiveness of coping strategies in terms of stress tolerance.

Values and beliefs

To assess the patient's values and beliefs, evaluate:
- cultural, sexual, and spiritual orientation
- goals and values that guide decisions.

Integrated and specialty database formats

For consistency, most health care facilities require that staff document assessment findings using standardized formats. Typically, history and physical findings are on the same form. The purpose of using a standardized format is to provide a comprehensive, consistent, understandable framework for nursing data. (See *The Joint Commission standards for initial assessments*.) Standardized formats enhance information exchange and communication among staff members and, when necessary, among health care facilities. However, when a standardized format is used, nurses typically adapt their assessment techniques to the flow of the form. Because most facilities use computerized documentation, nurses typically enter their assessment findings directly into a computer. (See *Integrated admission database form*, pages 42–47.)

Custom or generic?

Some facilities use assessment forms customized for their particular needs; others use more generic forms developed by outside vendors. These forms can be downloaded from the vendor either free or for a fee, depending on the vendor. Some standardized forms are designed to promote closer monitoring and evaluation of patient status trends, patterns, and longitudinal observations and changes. They're especially useful in critical care areas, where the patient's status can change in mere moments.

(*Text continues on page 47.*)

Memory jogger

To remember Gordon's functional patterns, think of the slogan "Hey Nurse! Every Action Can Start, Stimulate, Stop, or Reverse your Care Victory!"

HNEACSSRCV

Health perception and management

Nutrition and metabolism

Elimination

Activity and exercise

Cognition and perception

Sleep and rest

Self-perception and self-concept

Sexuality and reproduction

Roles and relationships

Coping and stress management

Values and beliefs

Weighing the evidence

The Joint Commission standards for initial assessments

The Joint Commission has developed standards for the initial nursing assessment of patients. The commission determines its standards by examining the criteria of nursing professional organizations and relevant research. The Joint Commission standards state that the following items should be considered in an initial assessment:
- physical factors
- psychological, social, and cultural factors
- environmental factors
- self-care capabilities
- learning needs
- discharge planning needs
- input from the patient's family and friends, when appropriate.

Integrated admission database form

Most health care facilities use a multidisciplinary admission form. The sample form below has spaces that can be filled in by the nurse, physician, and other health care providers.

MR No. 12345678 **Visit: 1234567891011** **Age: 36 (03/17/1976)**	**Holly Smith** **Female**	**ABC Hospital** **12 West**

General Information
- Language assistance needed? — No
- Source of information — Patient
- Arrived from — Home
- Valuables? — Yes
- Type of valuables — Cell phone, earrings, rings, and tongue and lip rings
- Disposition of valuables — With patient

Advance Directive
- Advance directive (medical health care) in place? — No
- Advance directive information given to patient — Living will brochure. Patient will notify staff if assistance is needed.
- Durable power of attorney in place? — No
- Is there anybody you would like to make medical decisions on your behalf in the event that you are unable to? — Nancy
- Relationship to patient — Mother

Spiritual Concerns and Care
- Are you part of a spiritual or religious community/congregation? — No
- Do you have any spiritual, religious issues/concerns? — No
- Do you consent to have your name appear on the spiritual care visitation listing? — Patient does not want spiritual or religious preference published or listed.

Allergies
- Fish — Reaction: Unknown
- Vancomycin — Reaction: Itching
- Doxycycline — Reaction: Undefined

Health and Illness
Current health and illness:
- Expected length of hospitalization — Unsure
- Primary care physician — Dr. Josephine Smith
- Services anticipated at discharge — None
- Anticipated discharge disposition — Home

Health and illness history:
- Previous general health — Average
- Previous healing pattern — Average
- Healing facilitated by — Rest
- Factors that prevent following health advice — None
- Health maintenance behaviors — Adequate sleep
- Previous reaction to anesthesia — None

Integrated admission database form (*continued*)

Height and Weight
- Actual height (ft):   5′
- Actual height (in): 3″
- Actual height (cm): 160 cm
- Actual weight (lbs): 141 lb
- Actual weight (kg): 64 kg
- Actual body surface area: 1.66 m^2
- Actual body mass index: 24.9 kg/m^2
- Actual weight 1 year ago: 154 lb

Nutrition and Metabolism
- Diet before admission (any restrictions, preferences)   Regular
- Current appetite   Fair
- Does patient have access to food?   Yes
- Who prepares meals?   Self
- Nutrition support   None
- History of eating disorder   None

Nutrition questions:
- Has patient lost more than 10 lb in the last 2 months without trying?   No
- Has patient been eating poorly over the last month, resulting in weight loss?   No
- Does patient have large or nonhealing wounds or pressure ulcers on admission?   No

Medication Information
- Medications brought to health care facility?   Yes
- Medication disposition   Sent home with family/friend

Roles and Relationships
- Significant relationships   Significant other
- Employment status   Currently employed
- Does patient provide primary care for anyone?   Children
- Limitations on visitors and phone calls   None

Living Environment
- Lives with   Significant other
- Living arrangements   Apartment
- Home accessibility concerns   None
- Financial concerns   None
- Available transportation   Car

Substance and Tobacco Use
Substance use: Current: Alcohol use
- Substance use   Past: Street drug/inhalant/medication abuse
- Alcohol type   Liquor
- Last alcohol use   2/14/12
- Duration of alcohol use (mo/yr)   Unsure

(*continued*)

Integrated admission database form (*continued*)

• Alcohol frequency	Monthly or less
• Alcohol amount	1–2 drinks
• Problems related to alcohol use?	No
Tobacco use:	Quit less than 1 year ago
• Tobacco use	6/23/11
• Date quit	10 menthol cigarettes/day × 14 years
• Tobacco form	Consistent exposure at home, in car, or at work
• Exposure to secondhand smoke	Less than daily
• Consistent exposure	Patient education folder provided; seen by smoking cessation
• Tobacco cessation information	Counselor
• Date seen	4/12/12

Systems Review

Neurologic:
• Neurologic conditions/symptoms	**None**

General pain information:
• Preferred pain scale	Numerical (0–10)
• Chronic pain?	No

Sleep and relaxation:
• Normal sleep/rest schedule	6–8 h/night
• Patient feels rested upon awakening?	Yes
• Any problem sleeping?	No
• Equipment/aids/routines for sleep	Watching television

Head, eye, ear, nose, and throat (HEENT):
• Dental care	Receives routine dental care
• Dental/oral status	Teeth intact, good condition
• Dentures?	No

Cardiac:
• Cardiac conditions/symptoms	None

Peripheral/neurovascular:
• Peripheral/neurovascular conditions/symptoms	None

Respiratory:
• Respiratory conditions/symptoms	Chest tube

Gastrointestinal:
• Gastrointestinal conditions/symptoms	None

Genitourinary:
• Genitourinary conditions/symptoms	None

Reproductive, female:
• Reproductive conditions/symptoms	None

Musculoskeletal:
• Musculoskeletal conditions/symptoms	Left rib fracture

Integrated admission database form (*continued*)

Mobility/activity:
- Ambulation: supervision/device needed   Independent
- Communication: issues/assistive device needed   None
- New or unaddressed problems   None

Home equipment:
- Any equipment used at home?   No

Previous level of functioning:
- Ambulation   (0) Independent
- Eating   (0) Independent
- Transferring   (0) Independent
- Toileting   (0) Independent
- Bathing   (0) Independent
- Dressing   (0) Independent
- Communication   (0) Understands/communicates without difficulty
- Swallowing   (0) Swallows foods and liquids without difficulty

Current level of functioning (if patient scored 2 or higher for any item, consult rehab services):
- Ambulation   (0) Independent
- Eating   (0) Independent
- Transferring   (2) Requires assistance
- Toileting   (1) Requires assistive equipment
- Bathing   (2) Requires assistance
- Dressing   (2) Requires assistance
- Communication   (0) Understands/communicates without difficulty
- Swallowing   (0) Swallows foods and liquids without difficulty

Skin:
- Skin conditions/symptoms   Piercing, tattoo
- Location of piercing(s)   Lip
- Location of tattoo   Lower back

Endocrine:
- Endocrine conditions/symptoms   None

Hematologic:
- Hematologic conditions/symptoms   None

Oncology:
- Oncology conditions/symptoms   None

Mental health:
- Mental health conditions/symptoms   Depression

Operations and procedures:
- Operation/procedure   Breast augmentation (2007)
- Operation/procedure   Computed tomography (7/10/10)
- Operation/procedure   Tonsillectomy (2005)

(*continued*)

Integrated admission database form (*continued*)

Self-Perception, Coping, and Stress Tolerance
Suicide risk:
- Is patient identified as a suicide risk?   No

Abuse screen:
- Have you ever been in a relationship where you have   Yes: emotional and physical
been threatened or abused physically, emotionally, or
sexually?
- Are you currently in a relationship where you are   No
threatened or abused physically, emotionally, or sexually?
- Do you feel unsafe going back to the place where you   No
live?
- Would you like to speak with a social worker/   No
counselor?

Learning Assessment
Patient:
- Education level   Completed high school
- Barriers influencing readiness to learn Acuteness of illness
- Factors impacting ability to learn   None
- Learning preferences   Individual instruction, verbal instruction
- Cultural considerations   None
- Developmental considerations   None
- Religious considerations   None
- Other learners   Significant other

Other learner:
- Learner   Significant other
- Education level   Quit high school after 10th grade
- Factors influencing readiness to learn   Acuteness of illness
- Factors impacting ability to learn   None
- Learning preferences   Individual instruction, verbal instruction, and skill
                                           demonstration
- Cultural considerations   None
- Developmental considerations   None
- Religious considerations   None

Mutuality/Individual Preferences
- Do you have any anxiety, fears, or concerns about   No
your health or care?
- Do you have any questions about your health care?   No
- Is there any information you can provide to help us   No
give you more personalized care?
- Verification: Mutuality statement reviewed and discussed with
                                                                patient, significant other, or family as appropriate to
                                                                ensure understanding
- What (if any) limitations would patient like on visitors,   None
television, or phone calls?

Integrated admission database form (*continued*)

Admissions Folder	
• Admission folder given to patient and/or family, as appropriate	Yes, reviewed with patient and/or family
• Instruction review code	(2) Meets goals/outcomes
• National Patient Safety Goals reviewed	Hand and respiratory hygiene, fall precautions
• Instruction review code	(2) Meets goals/outcomes
Electronic signatures:	**Stephanie Stellato, RN (Signed 4/15/12 0800)**

Digital age

Most health care providers use computerized charting to collect and organize real-time (or near real-time) patient information from various monitors. As a nursing student, you're probably familiar with these devices in other settings but expect to need time to adapt to integrating usage of these devices into your patient care.

Fancy formats

Narrative documentation used to be the primary means of recording data. However, formats, such as SOAP charting (subjective data, objective data, assessment data, and plan), SBAR charting (situation, background, assessment, recommendation), problem-oriented charting, and flow sheets, have become more common.

Exceptional charting

Computerized documentation often uses charting by exception. This type of charting calls for the nurse to record notes only on abnormal systems or issues. Each facility defines the guidelines to charting, which may include checklists, definitions of "normal," and the necessity for narrative supplements. Follow the guidelines set by your facility to correctly document nursing care and assessments.

Specialty assessments

Your patient's age and health status may require you to perform a more specialized examination. Specialty assessment tools include the Glasgow Coma Scale, pain rating scales, Mini-Mental Status Examination, and Dubowitz Gestational Age Assessment. The most common special assessments are those used for special populations, such as pediatric, elderly, maternal, and psychiatric patients.

You: the indispensable tool

Although standardized formats, specialty forms, and computerized data collection enhance and promote information collection and health care delivery, you—the nurse—are the primary collector of patient data. No matter what format your facility uses, data gathering and interpretation remain largely nursing responsibilities.

As a nurse, you're the ultimate—and indispensable—assessment tool. Not even the most sophisticated data collection tool or device can replace assessment by a skilled nurse.

Identifying growth and development stage

As children grow, they develop intellectually, morally, emotionally, sexually, socially, and spiritually. They learn to think abstractly and logically, use language, and explore the world around them. However, some theorists posit that growth and development don't end with childhood.

Erik H. Erikson is one of several theorists who explained how growth and development occur across the life span. As part of your assessment documentation, your instructors may ask you to identify which developmental stage your patient's growth represents. Although Erikson specifies an age range for each stage, don't be afraid to question whether your patient actually resembles a person facing the issues described. Some individuals may be mature beyond their years, while others may never have resolved the main crisis of a previous stage. Remember that you must be able to state why you believe your patient is moving through a particular stage. However, you aren't expected to be an expert in this area because you're still building your observation, listening, and communication techniques. Becoming familiar with Erikson's theory though will help you identify and better understand your patient's psychosocial needs and may be helpful in planning a teaching strategy.

Eight is enough

According to Erikson, psychosocial development occurs in eight distinct stages, which he calls "the eight stages of man." During each stage, a specific conflict occurs that the person must resolve. To resolve the conflict, the person undergoes a personality change, which gives him the strength to deal with the next developmental stage. If he can't resolve a conflict at a particular stage, he'll confront it later in life.

Stage 1: Trust vs. mistrust

During the first stage, which occurs from birth to about age 1, children develop trust if their needs are met. If their needs aren't met—or are met unpredictably—they become mistrustful.

Stage 2: Autonomy vs. shame and doubt

The second stage occurs between ages 1 and 3, when children learn to control their body functions and become increasingly independent. During this stage, they prefer to do things themselves and learn autonomy largely by imitating others. If they aren't allowed to be independent or are belittled for their efforts, they develop a sense of shame and self-doubt.

Did you know that the human head weighs 8 lb?

My assessment is that you're wise beyond your years.

Stage 3: Initiative vs. guilt

During stage 3, which occurs between ages 3 and 6, children learn about the world through play and learn to cooperate with others. They develop a conscience and learn to balance their sense of initiative against the guilt they experience for doing something against their parents' wishes. If they fail this developmental stage, as adults, they may be immobilized by guilt and continue to depend unduly on others.

Stage 4: Industry vs. inferiority

During stage 4, which occurs between ages 6 and 12, children enjoy working on projects and working with others. They tend to follow rules and become competitive. Social relationships take on great importance. If unrealistic expectations (or what they perceive as unrealistic expectations) are placed on them, they may develop feelings of inferiority. However, if they develop a sense of industry, they'll feel competent to meet life's expectations.

Stage 5: Identity vs. role confusion

From ages 12 to 18, adolescents experience rapid changes in their bodies. During this stage, they're preoccupied with how they look and how others view them. While trying to meet their peers' expectations, they also try to establish their own identity. If they fail to accomplish these tasks, they can suffer role confusion. If they navigate this stage successfully, they become confident adults who feel comfortable with who they are.

Stage 6: Intimacy vs. isolation

During this stage, young adults (ages 18 through 40) seek mutually satisfying relationships, including friends and marital partners. Many of them start families. Those who negotiate this stage successfully can experience intimacy on a deep level. Those who fail to do so become isolated and distant from others. Eventually, they may withdraw socially.

Stage 7: Generativity vs. self-absorption

During middle adulthood (ages 35 to 65), work and family take on great importance. People tend to be occupied with meaningful and creative work. They strive to contribute to the betterment of society and community, to transmit cultural values through the family, and to establish a stable environment. As their children leave the home or their relationships or goals change, major life changes may occur and they struggle to find new meanings and purposes (commonly referred to as a *midlife crisis*). Failure to negotiate this stage successfully can lead to self-absorption and stagnation.

Stage 8: Integrity vs. despair

During late adulthood (ages 65 to death), people look back on their lives and accomplishments. If they have found a meaningful role in life, have a positive self-concept, and can be intimate without strain, guilt, or regret, they have a feeling of integrity. On the other hand, those who despair at their experiences and perceived failure may fear death as they struggle to find purpose in their lives.

Integrating assessment into caregiving tasks

The key to accomplishing multiple responsibilities in a short time is to view all patient care tasks as opportunities to uncover critical information. Every contact you have with a patient gives you an opportunity for assessment. Crucial information may come to light even during seemingly insignificant interactions. Answering the call light, assisting with bathing, helping with range-of-motion exercises, and even making casual conversation during treatments and medication administration, these are all chances to observe the patient and gather valuable information.

> Remember that routine caregiving tasks provide an opportune time to collect valuable assessment data.

Example

Suppose, for example, that you're beginning your shift assignment. One of your patients is a 45-year-old woman who was admitted for cholecystectomy. The nurse presenting the change-of-shift report notes that the patient has been demanding and has been continually pressing the call light. The patient's chart indicates that her vital signs have been stable, she has reported good pain control, and she shows no signs of postoperative complications.

Dig deeper

Instead of simply accepting the "demanding" label used by the exasperated nurse on the previous shift, you decide to investigate the patient's condition and seek more information, suspecting that the patient's behavior could signal something deeper. Instead of waiting for the patient to press the call light, you take the initiative to check on her frequently. Over the next 2 hours, the patient appears to become more relaxed.

You decide to use the opportunity of morning care to spend a little extra time with the patient and assess her emotional and psychological status. As the patient washes her face and upper body, you stand quietly by her side. After a few moments, you ask her how she feels about her recent surgery and her recovery so far. She confides that she's been upset with her care in the hospital and also doesn't know how she'll manage at home. She begins to talk about all the problems she's had since the gallbladder attack just before admission. You listen carefully as the patient finishes washing, interjecting occasionally to show her that you're paying attention. As you begin massaging her back with lotion at the end of the bath, the patient tearfully reveals that her husband passed away several weeks ago—important information about the patient that you didn't previously know. During the seemingly routine chore of bathing, you have obtained information that could prove crucial to the patient's recovery and follow-up care—information that could help you to create a more appropriate care plan for this frightened, grief-stricken patient.

Data uncovered

As you can see from the previous example, taking time to assess the patient as you perform other caregiving tasks can help you to build rapport and uncover important patient information that may be crucial to your care plan.

Starting a concept map based on assessment data

During nursing education, you gain a tremendous amount of knowledge. But do you wonder how to put this theoretical knowledge into practice, especially when you have to care for more than one or two patients? Do you wonder how to start a care plan from your assessment data? Let's look at a possible scenario.

Example

You're a senior nursing student in your final rotation at a small community hospital. You're assigned to three patients on the medical-surgical unit. But before you can take vital signs on your patients, you learn you'll be receiving a pediatric patient from the ED because the pediatric unit is full. You look at your clinical instructor, hoping that she'll step in to change your assignment. Instead, she explains that the acuity level in the hospital has changed and that this will be a good opportunity for you to explore your clinical skills. Two of your other three patients are reassigned to other nurses.

The pediatric patient from the ED, John Scott, arrives within minutes. You observe that he's anxious, crying, and clinging to his mother, Christine Scott. The ED nurse gives the following report:

The child is an 8-year-old male who has had a high fever and severe stomach pain for the last 8 hours; abdominal guarding is present. Vital signs include temperature 101.6°F, heart rate 124 beats/minute, respiratory rate 28 breaths/minute, and blood pressure 132/80 mm Hg. Complete blood count and blood chemistry samples have been sent to the laboratory, along with a urine specimen for urinalysis. The patient is scheduled for an emergency exploratory laparoscopy within the hour to rule out a ruptured appendix.

You note that the boy's mother seems shaken and holds her child closely. Before leaving, the ED nurse takes you aside and tells you the mother is worried about the financial impact of this unexpected surgery. She hands you the patient's chart and leaves.

Don't push the panic button!

You're already running behind with your other patient. How can you possibly fulfill your nursing responsibilities to her and to your new pediatric patient? You need to admit the pediatric patient, introduce him to the hospital environment, assemble his chart, carry out the practitioner's admitting orders, verify that the necessary consents have been signed, make sure that the laboratory test results are back, and prepare the child (and his mother) for surgery. What's more, you need to perform an initial nursing assessment and then organize and document your findings before the boy goes to surgery so you can begin to develop a care plan. That's a tall order for a nursing student—or for *any* nurse. How would you handle it?

When asked to a panic party, turn down the invitation!

Chances are, you would feel overwhelmed, and your mind would race with frantic thoughts, such as: "Yikes! I have way too much to do and not nearly enough time to do it! So much is expected of me—and so fast. How can I meet all these demands and still make sure that my other patient is safe and receives good care?"

Serenity now

Remember not to panic. You're only human and can't possibly do everything at once. Before you can attend to your duties, you must attend to yourself, so take time to calm down and collect yourself. One way to do this is to stop, look, and listen. As a child, you were probably taught to stop, look, and listen before crossing a street.

The same procedure can help you focus when you find yourself in a stressful patient care situation. In this case, you stop first and then analyze what you've already looked at and listened to.

Stop sign

STOP stands for:
- **S**low down—Anxiety causes the release of adrenaline, a natural stimulant. (More stimulation is the last thing you need now!)
- **T**ake some deep breaths—However, many it takes to calm down.
- **O**bjectify your feelings—That is, treat them impersonally; you don't have to deny them, but you can choose to not let them control your actions.
- **P**repare a plan and proceed professionally.

After you accomplish the first three steps, the last one will be much easier. A plan gives you structure and direction and can be especially reassuring when you're feeling stressed out.

You know more than you know

Once you "stop" as described above, you'll find you feel less anxious, more in charge, and better able to think like a professional. Now, you're ready to analyze and organize the information you've already looked at and listened to—namely, the impressions you started to form from the time you met the patient and his mother and heard the ED nurse's report. That's right—you've been gathering assessment information without really being aware of it.

Let's look at what you know so far:
- The child is 8 years old.
- He has a high fever and is in pain.
- He has just been introduced to the strange sights, sounds, smells, and people in the hospital and has just heard people talking about him rather than to him.
- He's old enough to understand what surgery is.
- He's emotionally upset, and his mother is upset as well.

As you begin your structured nursing assessment, you'll build on the developmental, emotional, physical, and social information you've already collected.

Taking time for a concept map: what a concept!

Even in a hectic situation such as this, you might quickly sketch a concept map for yourself to help you focus on what you know and what you need to know. Utilizing just the data you've been given and what you've observed, you can rough out a concept map. (See *Getting started.*)

After you've gathered the patient assessment data, you're ready to move to the next step of the nursing process—formulating nursing diagnoses. As you learned in Chapter 1, creating a concept map helps you organize your thinking and see the big clinical picture.

Getting started

Begin your concept map for the pediatric patient described in text by placing a circle in the center of the page. In that circle, include the patient's name, age, and medical diagnosis. Also note that his mother is present, and include her name.

When you have little information but you need a plan quickly, don't try to formulate nursing diagnoses for your concept map right off the bat. Instead, jot down main categories of problems as you think of them. For example, you might start by labeling a box "GI symptoms" because you don't have enough information to get a handle on which nursing diagnoses are most appropriate. Include in this box any assessment findings that you collected from your observations and the shift report. Feel free to use abbreviations in your concept map (as shown below) to save time. Also, leave the boxes open so that you can add more information as you assess the patient and get his test results. You might not even want to draw connecting lines right away, but try to visualize the interrelationships in your mind.

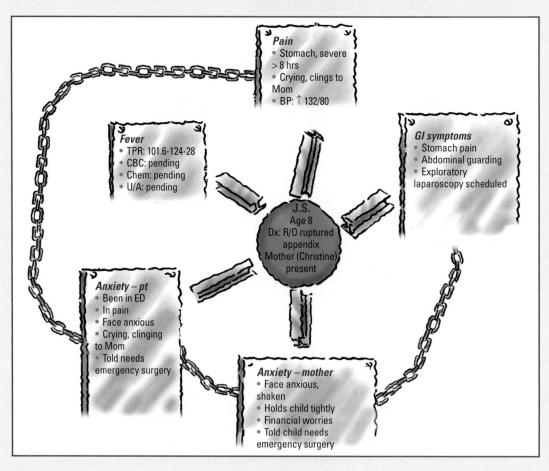

Pain
- Stomach, severe > 8 hrs
- Crying, clings to Mom
- BP: ↑ 132/80

Fever
- TPR: 101.6-124-28
- CBC: pending
- Chem: pending
- U/A: pending

GI symptoms
- Stomach pain
- Abdominal guarding
- Exploratory laparoscopy scheduled

J.S.
Age 8
Dx: R/O ruptured appendix
Mother (Christine) present

Anxiety – pt
- Been in ED
- In pain
- Face anxious
- Crying, clinging to Mom
- Told needs emergency surgery

Anxiety – mother
- Face anxious, shaken
- Holds child tightly
- Financial worries
- Told child needs emergency surgery

On the case

Case study background

Benny Hayes, a 38-year-old male, was brought to the emergency department (ED) after being involved in a boating accident. According to friends, he suffered a brief loss of consciousness at the scene. They report that he has a history of asthma. On admission, Mr. Hayes was groggy but easily aroused, scoring a 13 on the Glasgow Coma Scale. He complained of blurred vision, but his pupils were equal and reactive to light and accommodation. Vital signs were stable. He presented with a 3.5-cm hematoma on his left, posterior temporal area and a deep laceration on his left forearm. A computed tomography (CT) scan with contrast of the head and X-ray of the left forearm were normal. His laceration was sutured and he was given 1 g IV cefazolin via a saline lock, as ordered. An indwelling urinary catheter was also inserted.

When you start your shift, you are assigned to Mr. Hayes. The night shift nurse reports that Mr. Hayes was admitted with a concussion. His Glasgow Coma Scale score is now 15, his speech is normal, and his pupils are equal and reactive to light and accommodation. He received 1,000 mg of acetaminophen for a headache at 6:10 a.m. His left forearm dressing is dry and intact.

As you are organizing yourself to start your care, the charge nurse tells you that Mr. Hayes' doctor has ordered removal of the indwelling urinary catheter and discontinuation of the saline lock in preparation for discharge. You decide to proceed with your morning assessment and complete the discharge paperwork before checking and carrying out these orders.

Critical thinking exercise no. 1

When questioned by your instructor, you give three reasons why you decided to keep the urinary catheter and saline lock in place until just before discharge. They are:

1. _____

_____

2. _____

_____

3. _____

_____

You review the chart and jot notes in concept map form, while starting to fill in the discharge sheet you'll be giving to Mr. Hayes.

Concept mapping exercise

Complete the concept map below, including the problem labels (titles for the various boxes), by integrating all of the assessment information you have so far on Mr. Hayes. Note that information from the chart review is already added for you.

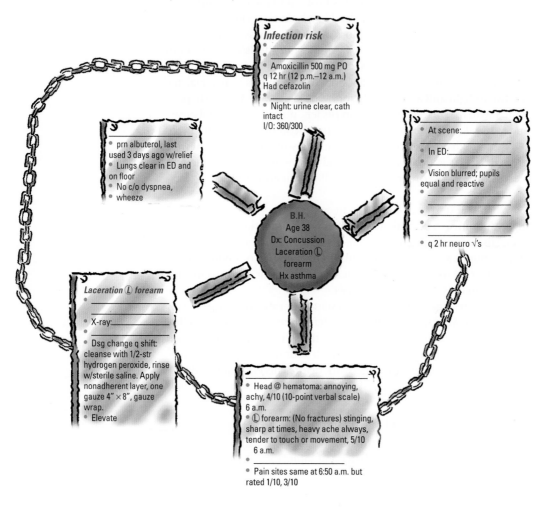

Infection risk
•
•
• Amoxicillin 500 mg PO q 12 hr (12 p.m.–12 a.m.) Had cefazolin
•
• Night: urine clear, cath intact
I/O: 360/300

• prn albuterol, last used 3 days ago w/relief
• Lungs clear in ED and on floor
• No c/o dyspnea,
• wheeze

• At scene:_____
• In ED:_____
•
• Vision blurred; pupils equal and reactive
•
• _____
• _____
• q 2 hr neuro √'s

B.H.
Age 38
Dx: Concussion
Laceration Ⓛ forearm
Hx asthma

Laceration Ⓛ forearm
_____
• X-ray:_____
•
• Dsg change q shift: cleanse with 1/2-str hydrogen peroxide, rinse w/sterile saline. Apply nonadherent layer, one gauze 4" × 8", gauze wrap.
• Elevate

• Head @ hematoma: annoying, achy, 4/10 (10-point verbal scale) 6 a.m.
• Ⓛ forearm: (No fractures) stinging, sharp at times, heavy ache always, tender to touch or movement, 5/10 6 a.m.
•
• Pain sites same at 6:50 a.m. but rated 1/10, 3/10

You return to Mr. Hayes' room to finish your assessment and redress the laceration on his left forearm. He's sitting up in a chair and you notice that he's sleepy and his speech is slower and less clear than it had been. Nonetheless, he reports, "I feel fine. I'm just waiting for breakfast."

Critical thinking exercise no. 2

1. The difference in Mr. Hayes' level of consciousness (LOC) may reflect:
   a. early morning hunger.
   b. beginning infection from the indwelling urinary catheter or arm wound.
   c. an increase in intracranial pressure (ICP).
   d. a normal variant in some individuals.
2. Your first action after seeing the change in Mr. Hayes is to:
   a. call the IV team to obtain a blood sample to send for a chemistry profile and complete blood count, while you obtain a urine sample for urinalysis with culture and sensitivity.
   b. take his vital signs, measure his pupils, check the remainder of his neurologic signs, and assist him into bed with the rails up.
   c. put up the bed rails, give him his call light, tell him to stay in bed, and then leave to find his primary nurse or your instructor to ask for assistance.
   d. apply oxygen and then call the practitioner immediately and request a repeat CT of the brain or magnetic resonance imaging of the brain because of a probable subdural hematoma.

Answer key

Critical thinking exercise no. 1

1. If Mr. Hayes' condition suddenly changed before discharge, an IV line might be needed for new medications.
2. If an untoward event occurs, the indwelling urinary catheter will be necessary to assess the patient's fluid balance.
3. You're responsible for fully assessing the patient so you can complete your portion of the discharge plan.

Concept mapping exercise

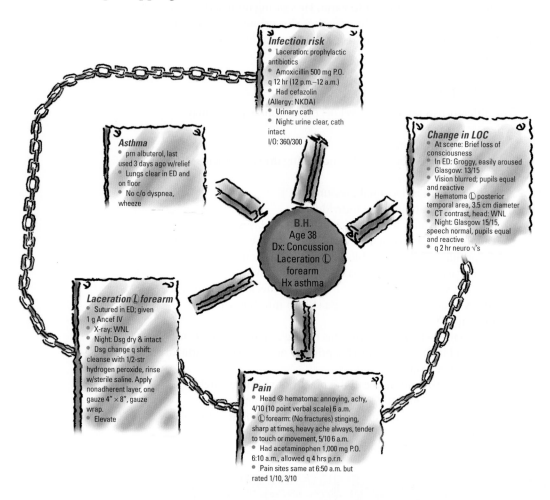

Infection risk
- Laceration: prophylactic antibiotics
- Amoxicillin 500 mg P.O. q 12 hr (12 p.m.–12 a.m.)
- Had cefazolin (Allergy: NKDA)
- Urinary cath
- Night: urine clear, cath intact
- I/O: 360/300

Asthma
- prn albuterol, last used 3 days ago w/relief
- Lungs clear in ED and on floor
- No c/o dyspnea, wheeze

Change in LOC
- At scene: Brief loss of consciousness
- In ED: Groggy, easily aroused
- Glasgow: 13/15
- Vision blurred; pupils equal and reactive
- Hematoma Ⓛ posterior temporal area, 3.5 cm diameter
- CT contrast, head: WNL
- Night: Glasgow 15/15, speech normal, pupils equal and reactive
- q 2 hr neuro √'s

B.H.
Age 38
Dx: Concussion
Laceration Ⓛ forearm
Hx asthma

Laceration Ⓛ forearm
- Sutured in ED; given 1 g Ancef IV
- X-ray: WNL
- Night: Dsg dry & intact
- Dsg change q shift: cleanse with 1/2-str hydrogen peroxide, rinse w/sterile saline. Apply nonadherent layer, one gauze 4″ × 8″, gauze wrap.
- Elevate

Pain
- Head @ hematoma: annoying, achy, 4/10 (10 point verbal scale) 6 a.m.
- Ⓛ forearm: (No fractures) stinging, sharp at times, heavy ache always, tender to touch or movement, 5/10 6 a.m.
- Had acetaminophen 1,000 mg P.O. 6:10 a.m., allowed q 4 hrs p.r.n.
- Pain sites same at 6:50 a.m. but rated 1/10, 3/10

Critical thinking exercise no. 2

1. C. A change in LOC is an early indicator of increased ICP. Hunger and early infection don't produce this sign. A subtle change in LOC is suspicious and may be the only early sign of increased ICP in a patient with a head injury. Pupillary changes are a later sign of increased ICP.

2. B. Because Mr. Hayes isn't in acute distress, your first action would be to assist him to a safer position in case of further deterioration; then, you would complete your neurologic check and vital signs assessment so you can give objective, useful information to the primary nurse or your instructor. Ordering laboratory work is out of

the scope of practice of the nurse. Making the patient safe is only a portion of your responsibility when a patient's status changes; a focused assessment of the new findings must also be completed unless the change is severe and beyond your skill level. There's no indication in the data given that the patient is in respiratory distress and may need immediate oxygen therapy. Independently calling a practitioner for orders is outside the scope of practice for a student.

Selected references

Ackley, B., & Ladwig, G. (2014). *Nursing diagnosis handbook: An evidenced-based guide to planning care* (10th ed.). St. Louis, MO: Elsevier-Mosby.

Assessment using functional health patterns. Retrieved on November 2016 from: http://www.delmarlearning.com/companions/content/0766822257/apps/appb2.pdf

Ballantyne, H. (2016). Developing nursing care plans. *Nursing standard, 30*(26), 51–57.

Classification of NANDA nursing diagnoses by Gordon's functional health patterns. Retrieved on November 2016 from: http://wcunurs120and121.pbworks.com/w/file/fetch/47889913/NANDA%20Gordon%20Functional%20Health%20Patterns.pdf

Erikson, E. H. (1993). *Childhood and society.* New York: WW Norton & Company.

Hinkle, J., & Cheever, K. (2014). *Brunner & Suddarth's textbook of medical-surgical nursing* (13th ed.). New York: Lippincott Williams & Wilkins.

Hockenberry, M., & Wilson, D. (2016). *Wong's essentials of pediatric nursing* (10th ed.). St. Louis, MO: Elsevier-Mosby.

Moattari, M., Soleimani, S., Moghaddam, N., & Mehbodi, F. (2014). *Clinical concept mapping: Does it improve discipline-based critical thinking of nursing students?* Retrieved on November, 2016 from: https://www.ncbi.nlm.nih.gov/pmc/articles/PMC3917188/

Nettina, S. (2014). *Lippincott's manual of nursing practice* (10th ed.). New York: Lippincott Williams & Wilkins.

Chapter 3

Nursing diagnosis

Just the facts

In this chapter, you'll learn:

◆ parts of a nursing diagnosis

◆ types of nursing diagnoses

◆ tips for identifying nursing diagnoses from concept map data.

A look at nursing diagnosis

Nursing diagnosis is the second step of the nursing process. After you've assessed the patient and clustered the findings into related areas, you must analyze these clusters to identify the patient problems that nursing care can address. Next, you'll create specific labels—nursing diagnoses—for each of your patient's problems.

A definition for the diagnosis

NANDA International (also called NANDA-I or NANDA, and formerly known as the North American Nursing Diagnosis Association) defines a nursing diagnosis as a "clinical judgment about an individual, family, or community response to actual or potential health problems or life processes which provides the basis for definitive therapy toward achievement of outcomes for which a nurse is accountable."

So what does this really mean? Let's break down this definition into digestible parts:

• A health problem is a circumstance such as illness, injury, or surgery or a lack of knowledge about a health issue.

• Life processes that can affect health include stressful events, such as divorce, pregnancy, or the illness or death of a loved one.

• Significant potential problems should also be addressed, such as risk for fall or risk for infection.

• The problem must be responsive to evidence-based, clearly outlined interventions.

• The nursing diagnosis must reflect a problem for which the nurse:

    ○ is legally permitted to intervene independently

    ○ can be held accountable for the outcomes.

Confused by NANDA's definition of a nursing diagnosis? You're not alone. At first glance, it can be a lot to swallow. But break it down into bite-size pieces, and it goes down easy!

To formulate nursing diagnoses, follow these steps:
1. Collect your assessment data, both subjective and objective findings.
2. Cluster the data that relate to specific problems.
3. Develop a problem list.
4. Prioritize your problem list.
5. Write a nursing diagnosis for each problem.

Suppose your patient reports shortness of breath while walking short distances, your assessment reveals nasal flaring, a rapid respiratory rate, and pursed-lip breathing. When clustering these data, you would see that these findings suggest a respiratory problem. Based on this, you would formulate an appropriate nursing diagnosis. Usually, your clustered data will lead you to establish several nursing diagnoses for each patient. You'll then arrange these diagnoses based on priority to ensure that you address the most crucial problems first.

Can't do without critical thinking

You'll need all your critical thinking skills to determine which nursing diagnoses are appropriate and to write diagnostic statements correctly. For example, understanding anatomy and physiology of the respiratory system and the way in which various lung disorders can alter respiratory function is critical to choosing between the nursing diagnoses *Impaired gas exchange, Ineffective airway clearance,* and *Ineffective breathing pattern.* If you select an inappropriate diagnosis, you're likely to choose ineffective nursing interventions, and your care plan will not only reflect your lack of understanding but will also fail to help the patient.

Do you like my new work? I call her the "Critical thinker." She's a favorite among nursing instructors.

Parts of a nursing diagnosis

A nursing diagnosis is commonly referred to as a *diagnostic statement* because its format includes all the information that a nurse would need to quickly understand the factors affecting a particular patient and the specific symptoms of his problem. An experienced nurse who's pressed for time could, therefore, provide appropriate care for the patient without even reading the expected outcomes and interventions listed on the care plan.

Nursing diagnoses can have three parts:
1. The first part is simply a **label**—for instance, *Readiness for enhanced parenting.* It describes an actual or potential patient problem that nursing care can influence. This part is usually written in NANDA-I–approved terminology.
2. Part two is the **etiology**, the related factors that precede, contribute to, or are associated with the patient's problem. Examples of related factors include diseases, injuries, birth defects, inherited

patterns, medical conditions, medical procedures, psychosocial factors, developmental phases, lifestyle, and situational or environmental factors. In the diagnosis, the etiology should be preceded by the words "related to," as in *Self-care deficit (bathing/hygiene) related to weakness*.

3. The third part of a nursing diagnosis is a list of the **signs and symptoms** that support the diagnosis. This part is preceded by the phrase **"as evidenced by**." For example, a three-part diagnosis for a psychiatric patient might read *Ineffective role performance (work) related to depression as evidenced by decreased concentration, increased daily sleep pattern, and frequent crying while awake*.

Memory jogger

When thinking about the three parts of a nursing diagnosis, remember that **LESS** is more. A nursing diagnosis that includes all three parts (NANDA-I Label, Etiology, and Signs and Symptoms) provides the most information about the patient's condition.

When to use which parts

You may notice that nursing textbooks, journals, and research papers sometimes refer to only one part of a nursing diagnosis (the diagnostic label) when defining patient problems. In some cases, the other two parts may be too specific for the discussion and are, therefore, unnecessary. In other cases, however, more detail is required, and the diagnosis may include the etiology as well.

The care plans that you write for school or in practice must include at least the first two parts of the diagnostic statement. Furthermore, if you're writing about a patient's existing problem, all three parts of the statement would be necessary for another nurse to understand the patient's situation. If the patient has the potential to develop a particular problem but has no current signs and symptoms, then the correctly written nursing diagnosis would contain just the first two parts of a diagnostic statement.

Types of nursing diagnoses

NANDA-I recognizes four types of nursing diagnoses:
- actual
- potential risk
- syndrome
- wellness.

Actual diagnosis

An actual nursing diagnosis describes an existing problem—a human response (individual, family, or community) to a health condition or life process that's validated by the presence of major defining signs and symptoms that cluster in patterns.

Everything's included

All three parts of a diagnostic statement are required for this type of diagnosis because:

- a NANDA-I label for the problem can be readily identified: *Ineffective infant feeding pattern* …
- the etiology can be specified: … *related to cleft palate…* (use the terms related to or due to)
- the patient exhibits qualifiable or quantifiable signs and symptoms of the response: … *as evidenced by the inability to form a mouth seal and abdominal distention from swallowed air.* (See *Adding evidence to the diagnosis.*)

Under construction

Adding evidence to the diagnosis

Writing a three-part nursing diagnosis is easy if you take it step by step. After writing the diagnostic NANDA-I term and the "related to" portion of the nursing diagnosis, add the evidence—findings that support the diagnosis you've chosen. Precede these findings with the words "as evidenced by." The evidence can be either subjective (such as the patient statement "I feel dizzy") or objective (such as vital signs or physical findings).

For example
For an otherwise healthy patient with an open arm fracture, you collect the following assessment findings:
- vital signs—temperature 98.9°F, pulse 104 beats/minute, respirations 20 breaths/minute, and blood pressure 124/76 mm Hg
- displacement of the humerus of the left arm, 6″ above the elbow
- ragged-edged wound at the site of the injury with localized bruising, swelling, and sanguineous oozing
- displaced fracture of the left humerus on X-ray
- facial grimacing and tearfulness
- pain rating of 6 on a 0 to 10 scale
- constant twitching and movement of the legs
- tight gripping of the side rail by the right hand
- patient statement, "I'm afraid of being put under for surgery. My aunt just died that way" (when told by the orthopedic surgeon that open reduction and internal fixation of the fracture is the best treatment for this injury).

Given the patient's statement regarding surgery, one of the nursing diagnoses you should choose is *Anxiety;* you add the etiology statement *related to fear of anesthesia*. Then, you should add the statement "as evidenced by" and choose only those assessment findings most pertinent to this particular diagnosis. Your list should include enough information to validate your choice of diagnosis but need not include every large and small piece of evidence you collected. In this example, you would complete your three-part diagnosis with *as evidenced by patient statement and stressful reaction regarding anesthesia for surgery.*

Potential risk diagnosis

A potential risk diagnosis describes a problem that the patient is *at risk* for developing. This type of diagnosis must:
- describe a problem or situation that could be prevented with proper planning and implementation of appropriate interventions
- be supported by risk factors (assessment data) that make the patient more vulnerable to the particular problem.

Risky business

The diagnostic label for a risk diagnosis always begins with the words *Risk for*. In addition, these diagnoses always contain only the first two parts of a diagnostic statement. Because the patient is just at risk for the problem, no signs and symptoms of the diagnosis are present (and therefore, you can't include an "as evidenced by" statement); you're simply developing a plan to prevent the problem from occurring. Say, for example, your patient has a fractured femur, is restricted to bed rest, and is obese. Based on these assessment findings, you might formulate a nursing diagnosis of *Risk for injury (thrombotic event or blood clot) related to obesity, decreased mobility, and bone fracture.*

Although the list of NANDA-I–approved diagnoses includes several risk diagnoses, you may also occasionally need to restate an actual diagnosis as a risk diagnosis if no other label appears appropriate.

Risk diagnoses are easy to identify; they begin with the words "Risk for."

Syndrome diagnosis

A syndrome diagnosis is a NANDA-I label specifically designed to serve as a shortcut in special diagnostic situations. A syndrome itself represents a pattern of signs and symptoms that, when found together, form a distinct clinical disorder. In medicine, many such syndromes have been identified—for example, Cushing's syndrome, acquired immunodeficiency syndrome, and fetal alcohol syndrome. In nursing, a syndrome diagnosis is used when a cluster of assessment findings or nursing diagnoses occur together, showing a specific clinical pattern. Syndrome diagnoses can be actual or potential risk diagnoses.

Six degrees of syndrome

Syndrome nursing diagnoses include a label, an etiology, and a group of signs and symptoms or nursing diagnoses. They always contain the word "syndrome" in the label. NANDA-I has approved six syndrome diagnoses:
- disuse syndrome
- impaired environmental interpretation syndrome
- posttrauma syndrome

- relocation stress syndrome
- rape trauma syndrome
- sudden infant death syndrome.

For example...

An individual with a nursing diagnosis of *Rape trauma syndrome* might appropriately be given multiple nursing diagnoses, such as *Acute confusion, Acute pain, Anxiety, Disturbed body image, Imbalanced nutrition: Less than body requirements, Insomnia, Powerlessness,* and *Sexual dysfunction.* However, a syndrome diagnosis can be used instead to provide a concise statement about the correlation among these factors and the rape event.

Even healthy people can be assigned nursing diagnoses. These diagnoses are called wellness diagnoses.

Wellness diagnosis

A wellness diagnosis describes a patient's response to a level of wellness. Typically, these diagnoses are used for patients who are already healthy but want to maintain or improve their wellness levels. These diagnoses are more commonly seen in clinics and other outpatient health care settings but can be used in any setting.

For example...

Suppose a 57-year-old male patient of normal height and weight with no history of medical problems wants to optimize his wellness by improving his diet and starting an exercise regimen. An appropriate wellness diagnosis might be *Readiness for enhanced self-health management related to knowledge about a regular exercise program.* Supporting data would include an existing wellness level and an expressed desire for optimal fitness and enhanced wellness.

Creating nursing diagnoses from a concept map

If you used a concept map to plot out your patient's assessment data, as described in Chapter 2, you can then use that map to help you define the best nursing diagnoses for your patient.

Example

As an example, let's expand on the case scenario used in Chapter 2 (page 52) You've settled the child and his mother into a hospital room and oriented them to the call light system and telephone usage. The child's and his mother's responses to your questions help you realize that they don't know what's involved in getting ready for surgery, what to expect after the surgery, or how long the surgery might last. The child is focused on his discomfort and points to the face labeled 8 on a 10-point faces pain rating card. He lies in the bed holding his abdomen, occasionally moaning, and complains of increasing nausea and head pounding. His skin is hot and dry, his color is pale, and he won't let you touch or listen to his abdomen. He hasn't experienced vomiting or diarrhea so far, and his last bowel movement was yesterday. His blood pressure is 126/74 mm Hg, temperature 102.4°F, pulse 120 beats/minute, and respirations 28 breaths/minute. His lungs are clear and all his peripheral pulses are intact.

Per the surgeon's orders, you initiate an IV line and start infusing dextrose 5% in normal saline solution. As you work, you explain to the child and mother what you're doing and why. You also explain that the surgeon wants the child to have a computed tomography (CT) scan of the abdomen before the procedure. You explain as simply as possible what a CT scan is. You also explain that the surgeon hasn't approved any pain medication because of the impending surgery (pain medication can mask important symptoms). When the child is transported to the CT scan department, you provide more information to the mother on the surgical process and care after the procedure. The pharmacy sends up the ordered dose of IV antibiotics preoperatively and you verify with the mother that the child has no known drug or latex allergies. You've already informed the surgeon of the mother's concerns about finances and obtained a referral for the social worker to visit. Per the mother's wishes, you've also notified the chaplain that she would like a visit as soon as possible.

With the above data in hand, you update your concept map, including the laboratory results that have returned. (See *Concept mapping for diagnosis,* page 67.)

Creating a problem list

When you develop a nursing diagnosis, you're translating the child's history data, physical findings, and laboratory data into a statement about his clinical status, responses to treatment, and nursing care needs. A good way to start is to use the assessment data you've gathered to develop a problem list, which describes the child's problems or needs. To help generate the list, you might want to prioritize the problems according to Maslow's Hierarchy of Needs (see page 81) and use Gordon's categories of functional health patterns (see page 37).

Problem child

In the problem list, identify the child's problems and needs with simple phrases, such as "high fever" or "GI distress." Then, look at the

Concept mapping for diagnosis

Now that you have more information, you can update your concept map by adding all the assessment data you've collected (as shown here in color) or just adding a few reminders based on the health assessment form you completed for admission.

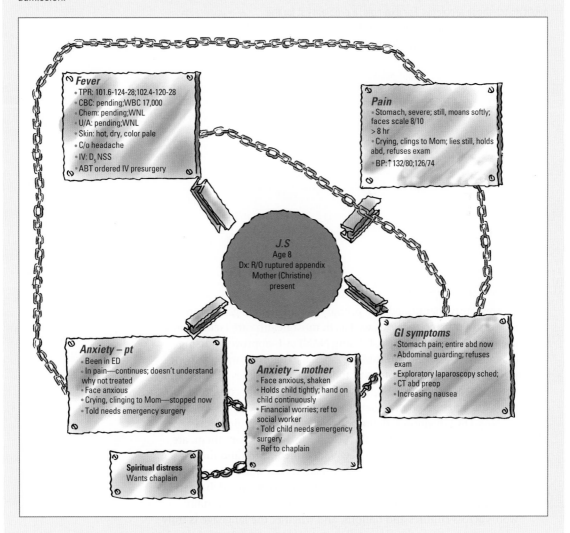

Fever
- TPR: 101.6-124-28;102.4-120-28
- CBC: pending;WBC 17,000
- Chem: pending;WNL
- U/A: pending;WNL
- Skin: hot, dry, color pale
- C/o headache
- IV: D$_5$NSS
- ABT ordered IV presurgery

Pain
- Stomach, severe; still, moans softly; faces scale 8/10
- >8 hr
- Crying, clings to Mom; lies still, holds abd, refuses exam
- BP: ↑132/80;126/74

J.S
Age 8
Dx: R/O ruptured appendix
Mother (Christine)
present

GI symptoms
- Stomach pain; entire abd now
- Abdominal guarding; refuses exam
- Exploratory laparoscopy sched;
- CT abd preop
- Increasing nausea

Anxiety – pt
- Been in ED
- In pain—continues; doesn't understand why not treated
- Face anxious
- Crying, clinging to Mom—stopped now
- Told needs emergency surgery

Anxiety – mother
- Face anxious, shaken
- Holds child tightly; hand on child continuously
- Financial worries; ref to social worker
- Told child needs emergency surgery
- Ref to chaplain

Spiritual distress
Wants chaplain

assessment data categories, such as activity exercise pattern or health maintenance pattern. For each category, determine if your patient is having a problem or is at risk for developing one. Then, formulate a tentative nursing diagnosis for each problem or potential problem. (See *Problems, problems list.*)

Problems, problems list

Once all of your assessment data are updated on your concept map, you can analyze these data to create a problem list. Find a corner on the map and list the problems you've noted. Then, begin to rough out the nursing diagnoses you believe might match those problems. For example, a problem list for the patient concept map at left might include the following problems and potential diagnoses.

PROBLEMS
- Fever, WBCs: Hyperthermia, Deficient fluid volume, Risk for infection
- GI sx: Ineffective protection; Risk for injury; Nausea; Risk for ineffective gastrointestinal tissue perfusion
- Pain: Acute pain
- Anxiety, mother: Anxiety, Spiritual distress, Stress overload, Compromised family coping

Writing a diagnostic statement

As previously mentioned, the primary nursing language used in schools of nursing today, as well as in most health care facilities and agencies, is that of NANDA-I. Using NANDA-I–approved nursing diagnoses, use a standard nursing language that confirms a patient problem, establishes etiology of the problem, validates the problem with evidence, justifies reimbursement of health care costs, and supports documentation of patient care.

NANDA-I diagnoses, definitions, related factors, and defining characteristics, as well as the taxonomy derived from them, are constantly changing to reflect newly identified needs and the latest research. NANDA-I meets every 2 years to review and revise existing nursing diagnoses and approve new ones. However, debate still continues on specific wording issues, appropriateness of certain words across cultures and nations, and whether the language is truly adequate to express the close collaboration between nurses and practitioners in managing and preventing disease complications.

Tale of the taxonomy

In 2000, NANDA-I changed its nursing diagnosis classification system from the original alphabetical listing, called Taxonomy I, to a conceptual system called Taxonomy II. The new system is based largely on Gordon's functional health patterns, but with some adjustments to reduce misclassifications and redundancies. (For more information on Gordon's functional health patterns, see page 37.)

Taxonomy II has three levels:

- domains
- classes
- nursing diagnoses.

Each domain includes several classes (refer to appendix NANDA-I Nursing Diagnoses by Domain pages 286–290). For instance, the self-perception domain has three classes—self-concept, self-esteem, and body image. Each class, in turn, has numerous approved nursing diagnoses. The self-esteem class of the self-perception domain, for instance, has three nursing diagnoses—chronic low self-esteem, situational low self-esteem, and risk for situational low self-esteem.

Differentiating the domains

NANDA International divides its 235 nursing diagnoses into 13 broad categories called *domains:*

- health promotion
- nutrition
- elimination and exchange
- activity/rest
- perception/cognition
- self-perception
- role relationships
- sexuality
- coping/stress tolerance
- life principles
- safety/protection
- comfort
- growth/development.

Dividing the domains

Each domain has up to six subdivisions called *classes.* The domain of *Health promotion,* for instance, has two classes—health awareness and health management. On the other hand, the *Safety/protection* domain has six classes—infection, physical injury, violence, environmental hazards, defensive processes, and thermoregulation. A total of 47 classes exist among the 13 domains.

Adapted from Herdman TH, Kamitsuru S. *Nursing diagnoses: Definitions and classification 2018–2020* (11th ed.). New York: Thieme. Copyright © 2018 NANDA International, Inc.

Wanted: new nursing diagnoses

NANDA International (NANDA-I) is seeking new nursing diagnoses to include in its taxonomy. Registered nurses are invited to submit new diagnoses they believe would be useful to their practice to NANDA-I's Diagnosis Development Committee (Diagnosis Review Committee). For details about submitting new diagnoses, visit www.nlinks.org or www.nanda.org.

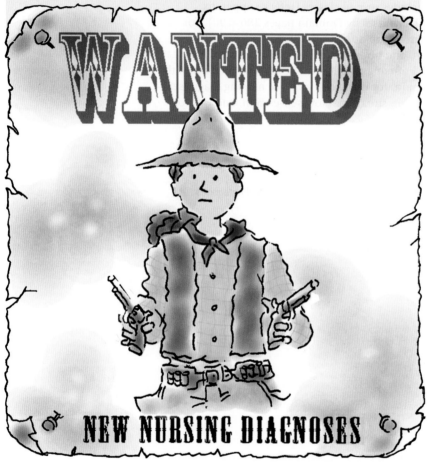

As of 2015, NANDA-I has approved a total of 235 nursing diagnoses where 26 of them are newly introduced and 16 are revised diagnoses. (See *Wanted: new nursing diagnoses,* above).

Dazed and confused

Some nurses have trouble writing nursing diagnoses because they find NANDA-I's terminology complex and the taxonomy confusing. Rather than listing diagnostic labels strictly alphabetically, NANDA-I lists the labels alphabetically "by diagnostic concept." However, nurses who aren't familiar with the concepts contained in the list can spend time searching for a label. For example, if a patient has bowel and bladder incontinence, you might reasonably think the major concept is incontinence and go to the letter I. However, "bowel" and "urinary" (not "bladder") are the diagnostic concepts that NANDA-I links to incontinence.

Another reason that NANDA-I can be difficult to use is that not all the problems you identify on your concept map can be readily found in NANDA-I terminology. Remember the boy with GI symptoms from Chapter 2? You might start looking for nursing diagnoses for this child under the letter "G" (for gastrointestinal), figuring that diagnoses related to stomach pain would be listed there. But you find none! Now what? Here's where critical thinking can be helpful.

Critically acclaimed

You apply your critical thinking skills by proposing these two questions to yourself and then answering them:

1. What type of physiology has been disrupted when severe abdominal pain and guarding and nausea are present? (*Answer:* Function of the GI tract)
2. At the simplest level, what patterns of function (NANDA-I domains) are presently most disrupted by this dysfunction within the GI tract? (*Answer:* Nutrition, activity and rest, coping and stress tolerance, safety and protection, and comfort). (See the appendix NANDA-I Nursing Diagnoses by Domain, pages 286–290.)

Making your list from NANDA-I terminology

Next, follow these six steps to identify the NANDA-I terminology that best describes your patient's problems:

1. Look over the diagnoses listed under "Nutrition." Because your patient is nauseated and cannot eat. The appropriate NANDA-I terminology is Imbalanced nutrition: Less than body requirements.
2. Move on to the "Activity and rest" domain. The diagnosis *Activity intolerance* catches your eye and you realize that this is one of your patient's problems. You add this NANDA-I terminology to your list.
3. Check the "Coping and stress tolerance" list. The diagnosis *Anxiety* heads this list, and you know that the child and mother are anxious at this time, although for different reasons. You jot down this NANDA-I term under the previous one.
4. Finish your search with the "Comfort" domain. You quickly realize that this domain yields two possible diagnoses: *Acute pain* and *Nausea*. You add them to your growing list of NANDA-I diagnostic terms.

Writing a nursing diagnoses in 3-part harmony

Now that you've chosen the NANDA-I diagnostic labels that best represent your assessment of the child's problems, you must complete the diagnostic statements. This means returning to your label list and filling in the second and third parts of each statement, as appropriate. The second part is the etiology of the problem. The third part is the evidence of the problem. For additional tips on writing nursing diagnoses the right way, follow the guidelines outlined in *The do's and don'ts of nursing diagnoses*, pages 72–73.

Under construction

The do's and don'ts of nursing diagnoses

Many nurses have trouble writing nursing diagnoses using NANDA International (NANDA-I) terminology. Some find the language complex, inadequate, abstract, vague, wordy, or clinically not useful. The following do's and don'ts may help you to muddle through the mass of NANDA-I's diagnoses to determine appropriate diagnoses for your patients. NANDA-I terminology is constantly scrutinized by nurses and the NANDA association always has new terminology on the "drawing board." NANDA-I is not a comprehensive list of every problem that can affect a patient. Therefore, some nursing educational programs and clinical settings accept other non–NANDA-I terminology in documentation.

Do
* Write diagnoses for problems that nurses are licensed to treat and that nursing interventions can resolve.
   ○ INCORRECT: *Uncontrolled blood pressure and recurrent gastroesophageal disease (daughter) related to mother's dependency on adult child for personal care as evidenced by mother's inability to be safe when alone and impaired functional capacity for personal hygiene*
   ○ CORRECT: *Caregiver role strain (daughter) related to mother's dependency on adult child for personal care and nurture as evidenced by mother's inability to be safe when alone and impaired functional capacity for personal hygiene*
* List the diagnostic label first and the medical cause (etiology) second.

   ○ INCORRECT: *Inadequate problem solving related to ineffective coping*
   ○ CORRECT: *Ineffective coping related to inadequate problem solving*
* Make the diagnosis clear and precise.
   ○ INCORRECT: *Ineffective community coping related to fear of their children catching meningitis from other school children who were close to the two girls who have meningitis as evidenced by the parents frequently keeping their children home from school and calling the practitioner to beg for antibiotics*
   ○ CORRECT: *Ineffective community coping related to acute meningitis outbreak as evidenced by decreased school attendance and markedly increased calls and visits to local health care providers*
* Include the diagnostic label, etiology, and signs and symptoms in all actual nursing diagnosis statements.

The do's and don'ts of nursing diagnoses (*continued*)

○ INCORRECT: *Moral distress as evidenced by patient's statements of belief in the sanctity of life from conception despite the recommendation for abortion to save the patient's life*

○ CORRECT: *Moral distress related to high risk of patient's death unless fetus is aborted as evidenced by patient's statements of belief in the sanctity of life at conception*

• Include only the diagnostic label and cause in all potential (*Risk for*) nursing diagnoses.

○ INCORRECT: *Risk for infection related to chemotherapeutic immune system suppression as evidenced by probable drug nadir in 10 days*

○ CORRECT: *Risk for infection related to chemotherapeutic immune system suppression*

Don't

• Write a diagnosis that focuses on a medical problem. (Nurses are only licensed to treat nursing problems.)

○ INCORRECT: *Heart failure related to acute myocardial infarction and atrial arrhythmia*

○ CORRECT: *Decreased cardiac output related to cardiac muscle death from a blood clot and atrial arrhythmia*

• Write a diagnosis that focuses on a nursing goal.

○ INCORRECT: *Promote early postoperative ambulation related to risk of prolonged immobility*

○ CORRECT: *Ineffective peripheral tissue perfusion related to prolonged postoperative immobility*

• Write a diagnosis that focuses on difficulty accomplishing a nursing intervention.

○ INCORRECT: *Difficulty administering tube feedings related to gastrostomy feeding tube insertion as evidenced by kinking of feeding tube*

○ CORRECT: *Imbalanced nutrition: Less than body requirements related to difficulty swallowing and initiation of feeding by gastrostomy tube*

• Create a diagnosis for a treatment or diagnostic test.

○ INCORRECT: *Ventilation-perfusion scan and computed tomography scan of the lungs with contrast related to risk of decreased tissue perfusion (respiratory)*

○ CORRECT: *Risk for decreased cardiac tissue perfusion related to postoperative immobility and minute thromboemboli seen on ventilation-perfusion scan*

• Say the same thing twice.

○ INCORRECT: *Total urinary incontinence related to unpredictable urine loss*

○ CORRECT: *Total urinary incontinence related to spinal cord injury as evidenced by inability to sense or contract the urinary sphincter*

Collaborative care

Not all nursing diagnoses can be managed solely by the nurse. To meet desired patient outcomes, some diagnoses require interprofessional collaborative management by the nurse with a physician, a nurse practitioner, a physician's assistant, a pharmacist, a dietitian, a social worker, a physical therapist, a clergyperson, or another health care professional. (See *Concerns about collaborative care*, page 74.)

Elaboration on collaboration

Interprofessional collaborative care encompasses the following:

• A health care practitioner, usually a physician or nurse practitioner, is responsible for ordering definitive treatments or tests.

• A staff nurse is responsible for implementing the orders, acting within the standard of care, monitoring the patient, and taking measures to prevent complications, as needed.

Concerns about collaborative care

Educational institutions, health care agencies, nursing professionals, and specialists on the language of nursing incorporate documentation of collaborative care within the nursing care plan in various ways.

Collaborative problem list

Lynda Juall Carpenito-Moyet, an expert on nursing diagnoses, has long advocated for care plans to include a "Collaborative Problem" category that describes physiological complications for which practitioners prescribe treatments but nurses monitor and carry out the medical and any related nursing interventions. She recommends that these problems be listed with the nursing diagnoses at the beginning of a nursing care plan and be preceded by the letters "PC," meaning "potential complication." Examples could include:

- PC: Bleeding
- PC: Pneumonia.

Nursing intervention labels

Other specialists in nursing language indicate that the collaborative nature of patient care is best reflected in the nursing interventions. Thus, they list interventions as "independent" or "collaborative." Independent nursing interventions are those that a nurse can implement for a patient that is within the scope of legal, standard nursing care.

For example, a patient who's experiencing hard stools while hospitalized may be assigned a nursing diagnosis of *Risk for constipation*. For this diagnosis, standards of nursing care would recommend such nursing interventions as providing the patient with adequate oral fluids, assisting the patient to ambulate in the hall twice per day, and teaching the patient the importance of choosing foods high in fiber. However, if the patient reports that he regularly used a stool softener at home, the nurse can initiate collaborative care interventions. This would include reporting these findings about constipation to the health care practitioner (physician or nurse practitioner) and recommending a prescription for a daily stool softener for the patient.

- A nurse may coordinate care with another health care professional, for example, a certified nursing assistant, to implement the care needed for the patient.

Most interprofessional collaborative care is necessary in patients with complex physiological conditions that require intensive monitoring and potential complications. Examples of proposed interprofessional collaborative care diagnoses might include:

- *risk of hypovolemic shock related to blood loss*
- *risk of postoperative complications*
- *risk of arrhythmia related to permanent pacemaker malfunction.*

Clearly, the above diagnoses cannot be managed by only a nurse. Many interprofessional members of the health care team must collaborate in the care of the patient with these diagnoses.

To complicate matters...

However, *not all* physiological complications call for collaborative diagnoses. Suppose your patient is developing a contracture due to lack of mobility, has a stage 1 break in skin integrity, or is at risk for an infection from an external source. In this case, the nurse can independently initiate and implement preventive measures. Thus, the problem is considered a nursing care issue for which a nursing diagnosis, nursing judgment, and independent nursing management are appropriate.

Create your own

NANDA-I acknowledges that not all potential nursing diagnoses, including some that relate to collaborative care, have yet been proposed or validated through their governing body. Therefore, most educational institutions allow students to include properly worded but non–NANDA-approved nursing diagnoses in their care plans. Some facilities label these diagnoses as "collaborative problems"; others handle these diagnoses in different ways.

The documentation of collaborative care concerns, as with other non–NANDA-I–approved diagnoses, remains at the discretion of the clinical or educational institution involved. This book focuses on the correct format of a nursing diagnosis and how to choose an appropriate NANDA-I nursing diagnosis. The issue of collaborative care is discussed again in the next chapter as it relates to expected outcomes and nursing interventions. (See *Choosing a NANDA-I diagnosis*, page 76).

Comparing nursing diagnoses and medical diagnoses

Once you become familiar with nursing diagnoses, you'll clearly see how nursing practice and medical practice differ. Both nurses and doctors identify patient problems, but they use different types of diagnoses and different treatment approaches. Medical diagnoses are more disease focused, whereas nursing diagnoses are more patient focused.

An interesting distinction

The main difference is that doctors are licensed to diagnose and treat a medical disease or condition, whereas nurses are licensed to diagnose and treat a patient's *response* to a disease or condition. So a nursing diagnosis describes a *response* to a disease—not the disease itself.

Here is an example of a medical diagnosis versus a nursing diagnosis in a patient with heart failure.

Medical diagnosis: Pulmonary edema secondary to congestive heart failure.

Nursing diagnosis for the same patient: Impaired gas exchange due to pulmonary edema as evidenced by dyspnea, orthopnea, and cough.

Choosing a NANDA-I diagnosis

What should you do if you can't easily identify a NANDA International (NANDA-I) diagnosis that applies to the patient problem you've identified? Use the algorithm below to help you.

If you have reanalyzed the data and are still convinced that *no* NANDA-I diagnosis is appropriate, consult with your instructor about using a *non–NANDA-approved* nursing diagnosis or a collaborative diagnosis.

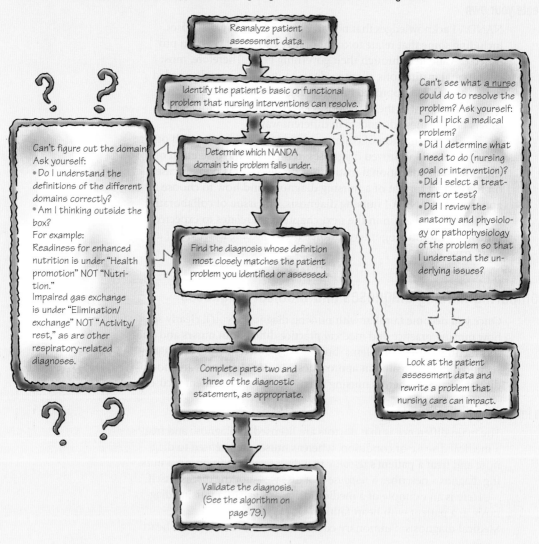

Reanalyze patient assessment data.

Identify the patient's basic or functional problem that nursing interventions can resolve.

Determine which NANDA domain this problem falls under.

Find the diagnosis whose definition most closely matches the patient problem you identified or assessed.

Complete parts two and three of the diagnostic statement, as appropriate.

Validate the diagnosis. (See the algorithm on page 79.)

Can't figure out the domain? Ask yourself:
• Do I understand the definitions of the different domains correctly?
• Am I thinking outside the box?
For example:
Readiness for enhanced nutrition is under "Health promotion" NOT "Nutrition."
Impaired gas exchange is under "Elimination/exchange" NOT "Activity/rest," as are other respiratory-related diagnoses.

Can't see what a nurse could do to resolve the problem? Ask yourself:
• Did I pick a medical problem?
• Did I determine what I need to do (nursing goal or intervention)?
• Did I select a treatment or test?
• Did I review the anatomy and physiology or pathophysiology of the problem so that I understand the underlying issues?

Look at the patient assessment data and rewrite a problem that nursing care can impact.

As you can see, the nursing diagnosis is based on how the patient is reacting to the disease and the symptoms that need to be addressed.

However, nursing diagnoses aren't limited to patients' responses to diseases. Nurses also can diagnose the need for:

- patient education
- comfort and counseling
- care until the patient is physically and emotionally capable of providing self-care.

Another notable difference

Another way in which nursing diagnoses differ from medical diagnoses is that nursing diagnoses may change frequently during a patient's hospital stay or during the recovery process. As a patient progresses through the stages of illness toward problem resolution, the nursing diagnoses you formulate for him are likely to change correspondingly. (See *Adapting to changes,* pages 77–78).

Remember, nurses treat the patient, not the disease. That important distinction is reflected in nursing diagnoses.

Adapting to changes

To illustrate the variability of nursing diagnoses versus the relative stability of medical diagnoses, consider the case of J.D., a 69-year-old retired carpenter with a medical history of hypertension and hyperlipidemia. He takes olmesartan and hydrochlorothiazide (Benicar HCT) 40/25 mg and simvastatin (Zocor) 20 mg daily. He's married to 64-year-old N.D., who works 40 to 50 hours/week and is the primary housekeeper, cook, and grocery shopper for the family. Follow his diagnoses through the course of an acute illness.

Course of the illness	Medical diagnoses	Nursing diagnoses
While his wife is at work, J.D. develops sudden, severe weakness in his right (dominant) arm and right lower lip, with milder weakness in the right leg. He calls 911 but can't relay to the responders what happened or a medical or drug history. He's confused to time and place and says anxiously, "I don't want to die." He's taken to the hospital, where a computed tomography scan shows no signs of cerebral hemorrhage or clotting, but his blood pressure is 192/108 mm Hg. J.D. is admitted.	Rule out: • Stroke • Hypertension • Hyperlipidemia	• *Risk for ineffective cerebral tissue perfusion related to hypertension and possible stroke* • *Risk for injury related to confusion and right-sided weakness* • *Fear related to sudden body changes and risk of death*
N.D. arrives at the hospital 5 hours later but stays for only 2 hours. Within these first few hours of admission, J.D. complains to the nurse about an inability to urinate. A bladder ultrasound shows 600 mL of urine in the bladder, and the nurse inserts an indwelling urinary catheter. J.D.'s urine culture is positive for infection, and antibiotic treatment is ordered. J.D.'s weakness and confusion don't progress, and his lip drooping disappears. His blood pressure decreases to 186/96 mm Hg. J.D. still expresses fear that "this is the end."	Rule out: • Stroke • Hypertension • Hyperlipidemia • Urinary tract infection (UTI)	• *Risk for ineffective cerebral tissue perfusion related to hypertension and possible stroke* • *Risk for injury related to confusion and right-sided weakness* • *Death anxiety related to sudden body changes and risk of death* • *Urinary retention related to UTI*

(continued)

Adapting to changes (continued)

Course of the illness	Medical diagnoses	Nursing diagnoses
Gradually, all of J.D.'s neurologic symptoms disappear, except for some residual disorientation to time. J.D. verbalizes understanding that his condition is treatable. After 3 days, J.D. and N.D. are informed that discharge is imminent, and the nurse assesses their ongoing care and learning needs. N.D. has visited J.D. only briefly each day and states she has little time to learn a new diet; J.D. says he can't remember it all. J.D. is discharged from the hospital with a referral for home care services due to ongoing concerns for home safety and health maintenance and the need for more teaching regarding blood pressure management.	• Transient ischemic attack (TIA) • Hypertension • Hyperlipidemia • UTI	• *Deficient knowledge (patient): Medication regimen related to new antihypertensive and anticlotting medications* • *Deficient knowledge (patient and wife): Low-salt, low-fat diet related to new diet orders* • *Risk for injury related to possible recurrence of TIA or stroke*
The home care nurse visits J.D. the following evening and completes an assessment. N.D. is present for the visit and expresses minimal willingness to learn about recommended dietary adjustments. She states: "I'm just too busy; I can't do it all. He needs to do more for himself and the house. He's gotten so lazy." J.D. also admits to not taking his medications regularly before the hospital admission.	• TIA • Hypertension • Hyperlipidemia	• *Deficient knowledge (patient and wife): Low-salt, low-fat diet related to new diet orders* • *Deficient knowledge (patient): Medication regimen and risk factors for stroke related to inadequate time for teaching due to patient's learning style (repetition and demonstration required)* • *Ineffective family therapeutic regimen management related to interspousal conflict over roles and skills* • *Risk for injury related to deconditioning during hospitalization, hypertension, and risk of stroke or TIA*
During the course of J.D.'s care, the home care nurse reports to the practitioner that the patient shows difficulty with short-term memory and has a Mini-Mental Status Examination score of 26 (indicative of early dementia). The practitioner orders a magnetic resonance image of the brain, which shows signs of multiple small infarctions. N.D. verbalizes more acceptance of J.D.'s caregiving needs and willingness to learn new skills when the testing shows he isn't deliberately refusing to be responsible.	• TIA • Hypertension • Hyperlipidemia • Multi-infarct dementia	• *Deficient knowledge (patient and wife): Multi-infarct dementia* • *Deficient knowledge (patient and wife): Low-salt, low-fat diet related to new diet orders* • *Impaired memory related to cerebral injury* • *Risk for injury related to deconditioning during hospitalization, hypertension, and risk for stroke or TIA*

Validating nursing diagnoses

After you have finished developing all of the patient's nursing diagnoses, you must go back and check each of the statements again to validate them. Determine the accuracy of assessment data, priority of the

Validating a diagnosis

You've completed all your nursing diagnoses statements. What's next? Validation of the diagnoses. Follow the rest of the algorithm on your path to understanding the trick to successful nursing diagnosis.

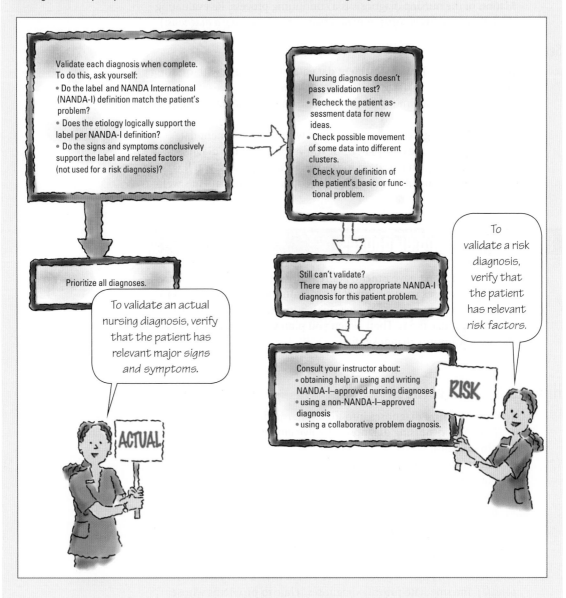

Validate each diagnosis when complete. To do this, ask yourself:

• Do the label and NANDA International (NANDA-I) definition match the patient's problem?
• Does the etiology logically support the label per NANDA-I definition?
• Do the signs and symptoms conclusively support the label and related factors (not used for a risk diagnosis)?

Nursing diagnosis doesn't pass validation test?

• Recheck the patient assessment data for new ideas.
• Check possible movement of some data into different clusters.
• Check your definition of the patient's basic or functional problem.

Prioritize all diagnoses.

To validate an actual nursing diagnosis, verify that the patient has relevant major signs and symptoms.

Still can't validate?
There may be no appropriate NANDA-I diagnosis for this patient problem.

To validate a risk diagnosis, verify that the patient has relevant risk factors.

Consult your instructor about:
• obtaining help in using and writing NANDA-I–approved nursing diagnoses
• using a non-NANDA-I–approved diagnosis
• using a collaborative problem diagnosis.

ACTUAL

RISK

problem list, NANDA-I diagnostic terminology, and evidence from the patient's signs and symptoms. Then, critically analyze your information from the patient's current status, verifying that the etiology accurately applies to the patient's condition and justified by the patient's signs and symptoms as evidence. The assessment data, nursing diagnosis, etiology, and evidence must be constantly validated and may need revision as the status of the patient changes. The practice of review and validation of the nursing diagnosis is a continuing process. Re-evaluating the patient's status is constantly necessary. (See *Validating a diagnosis.*)

Searching for support

If most of the patient's assessment data aren't consistent with or don't support the nursing diagnosis, you can either:
- reassess the patient for additional assessment data that *do* support the diagnosis
- revise the diagnosis so it's consistent with the assessment data.
  Don't initiate the care plan until you've validated the diagnoses. If you write a care plan based on invalid nursing diagnoses, you'll waste time implementing it—and you could jeopardize your patient's well-being.

Prioritizing nursing diagnoses

Usually, you won't have time to address all—or even most—of the nursing diagnoses you've formulated for your patient. You'll need to focus on the most important ones, which means that you'll have to be able to prioritize them. Then, when you plan your care, you address the highest-priority diagnoses first.

High, low, and in between

You can prioritize diagnoses into high, intermediate, and low priority:
- *High-priority* nursing diagnoses involve emergency or immediate physiological needs.
- *Intermediate-priority* diagnoses involve nonemergency needs or potential risks.
- *Low-priority* diagnoses involve needs that don't directly relate to the patient's current illness or recovery. These are often patient care needs that require a long-term plan.
  For example, for an acute care patient in a nonpsychiatric setting, high-priority nursing diagnoses typically relate to airway, breathing, and circulation (e.g., *Decreased cardiac output related to cardiac tamponade*). Intermediate-priority diagnoses relate to problems whose resolution can impact the patient's speed or degree of recovery but

The power of Maslow's pyramid

Maslow's pyramid can help you prioritize a patient's nursing diagnoses. Physiological needs—represented by the base of the pyramid in the diagram below—must be met first.

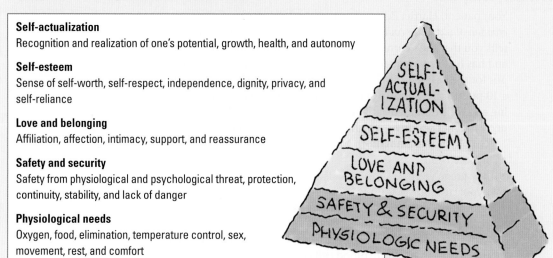

Self-actualization
Recognition and realization of one's potential, growth, health, and autonomy

Self-esteem
Sense of self-worth, self-respect, independence, dignity, privacy, and self-reliance

Love and belonging
Affiliation, affection, intimacy, support, and reassurance

Safety and security
Safety from physiological and psychological threat, protection, continuity, stability, and lack of danger

Physiological needs
Oxygen, food, elimination, temperature control, sex, movement, rest, and comfort

aren't life-threatening (e.g., *Risk for infection related to indwelling urinary catheter*). Low-priority diagnoses commonly address anxiety, fear, self-esteem, or a preexisting chronic problem to which the patient has adapted (e.g., *Insomnia related to variable shift work schedule as evidenced by sleeping during the day, awake at night since hospitalized*).

Prioritizing props

You can use the problem list you created to help you prioritize nursing diagnoses, or you can refer to Maslow's Hierarchy of Needs. This hierarchy classifies human needs based on the concept that physiological needs must be met before more abstract needs can be addressed. (See *The power of Maslow's pyramid*.)

Out of time

You might need to provide a referral to the patient at discharge to help him manage ongoing recovery or long-term impairment, problems that a nurse in an acute care setting can't fully address. If you are working in a rehabilitation facility, skilled nursing facility, inpatient psychiatric center, or home health care agency, your care plan should address the long-term needs and concerns of the patient.

Maslow's pyramid can help you prioritize nursing diagnoses.

On the case

Case study background

Your patient, Harriet Zoose, has a medical diagnosis of *Acute exacerbation of ulcerative colitis*. When you obtain her health history, she tells you that she's currently experiencing painful abdominal cramps and has had very frequent bowel movements containing blood and pus for the past few days. She rates her discomfort level at a 7 on a 10-point scale. She also states she has recently had trouble sleeping and feels extremely fatigued. She says the colitis has drastically decreased her sex drive, which is causing tension within her marriage.

On physical examination, you assess:

- hypotension
- low-grade fever
- hypoactive bowel sounds
- abdominal distention and tenderness
- pallor.

When you review her diagnostic data, you note that she has a moderately elevated white blood cell count; slightly elevated blood urea nitrogen (BUN) level; decreased hemoglobin level, hematocrit, and total protein level; and a prolonged bleeding time. An upper GI series performed the previous day found scarred and stenotic bowel segments, which are obstructing the intestinal flow.

Critical thinking exercise

Together, the nursing and medical diagnoses—and the care plan overall—should describe the complete nursing care the patient needs. For this patient, the care plan should include nursing diagnoses that address her *response* to her medical diagnoses. List four three-part nursing diagnoses for this patient. (Note that there are more than four correct answers.)

1. _____
_____
_____

2. _____
_____
_____

3. _____
_____
_____

4. _____
_____
_____

Answer key

Here are some examples of nursing diagnoses that could be appropriate for this patient:

1. *Deficient fluid volume related to acute diarrhea and blood loss as evidenced by decreased hemoglobin level and hematocrit, increased BUN level, and decreased blood pressure*
2. *Risk for infection related to potential bowel perforation and general debilitation*
3. *Chronic pain related to abdominal cramping and distention as evidenced by pain scale rating and patient statements*
4. *Insomnia related to anxiety and uncomfortable sensations as evidenced by patient statements*
5. *Ineffective sexuality pattern related to decreased physical energy and chronic, uncomfortable physical symptoms as evidenced by decreased sexual interest per patient statements*
6. *Fatigue related to decreased hemoglobin level and hematocrit, pain, and exacerbation of colitis as evidenced by patient statements and decreased hours of sleep*
7. *Interrupted family processes related to increased symptoms of ulcerative colitis as evidenced by patient complaints of decreased libido and resultant marital tension*

Selected references

Ackley, B., & Ladwig, G. (2014). *Nursing diagnosis handbook: An evidence-based guide to planning care* (10th ed.). Maryland Heights, MO: Mosby Elsevier.

Ballantyne, H. (2016). Developing nursing care plans. *Nursing Standard, 30*(26), 51–57.

Continuing Professional Development. (2015). *Developing nursing care plans*. Retrieved on November 2016 from: http://journals.rcni.com/doi/pdfplus/10.7748/ns.30.26.51.s48

Herdman, T. H., & Kamitsuru, S. (2018). *NANDA International, Inc. Nursing diagnoses: definitions & classification 2018–2020* (11th ed.). New York: Thieme.

Hinkle, J. L., & Cheever, K. H. (2014). *Brunner & Suddarth's textbook of medical-surgical nursing* (13th ed.). Philadelphia, PA: Wolters Kluwer.

Jalil, E. R. (2016). *NANDA nursing diagnosis list 2015–2017*. Retrieved on November 2016 from: http://health-conditions.com/nanda-nursing-diagnosis-list-2015-2017/

Lewis, S. L., Bucher, L., Heitkemper, M. M., & Harding, M. M. (2017). *Medical-Surgical nursing: Assessment and management of clinical problems* (10th ed.). St. Louis, MO: Saunders.

NANDA International. *How do I write a diagnostic statement for risk, problem-focused and health promotion diagnoses?* Retrieved on December 2016 from: http://kb.nanda.org/article/AA-00492/36/English-/Frequently-Asked-Questions/Nursing-Diagnosis/Nursing-Diagnosis%3A-Learning-Using/How-do-I-write-a-diagnostic-statement-for-risk-problem-focused-and-health-promotion-diagnoses.html

Nettina, S. (2014). *Lippincott's manual of nursing practice* (10th ed.). New York: Lippincott Williams & Wilkins.

Chapter 4

Planning

Just the facts

In this chapter, you'll learn:

◆ skills for developing and writing measurable, achievable patient outcomes

◆ factors that influence behavior and contribute to patient adherence to the plan of care

◆ classifications of nursing interventions

◆ guidelines for developing and writing effective nursing interventions

◆ the relevance of evidenced-based practice in planning care.

Care plan components

After you establish and prioritize a patient's nursing diagnoses, you're ready to identify patient outcomes and develop a written care plan. Recall that the nursing care plan is a written plan of action designed to help you deliver quality patient care. It is based on the problems identified during patient interview and includes these three major components:

• nursing diagnoses
• expected outcomes
• nursing interventions.

One size doesn't always fit all

Care plans may be traditional (plans that are created from scratch) or standardized (preprinted plans that can be tailored to a patient's individual needs). As a student, you'll most likely use some form of traditional care plan format designed by your faculty until you've gained more experience in critical thinking. You may be instructed to use this care plan in conjunction with concept mapping. During your clinical rotations, you'll consult the care plan tool used by the individual facility. Keep in mind that a patient's problems and needs can change, so you'll need to review the care plan often and modify it as necessary.

Writing the care plan for a patient really starts with planning achievable goals with the patient and deciding the best ways to reach them. Gathering assessment data and developing nursing diagnoses form the basis for this plan.

Take three giant steps

Writing an initial care plan involves these three steps:
- reviewing the established diagnoses and assessment data if needed
- identifying expected patient outcomes and specific nursing interventions to attain those outcomes
- documenting the nursing diagnoses, expected outcomes, and nursing interventions in a clear, consistent format.

The first step above was covered in detail in the previous chapters. It is included here as a reminder that you should know your patient's established diagnoses and current status before you begin planning specific care needs.

Tailoring a standardized care plan to each patient guarantees the best fit.

Identifying expected patient outcomes

During outcome identification, you must focus on determining appropriate goals, or expected outcomes, for a patient based on the nursing diagnoses you've already formulated. Remember, the ultimate goal of your nursing care is to help the patient reach his highest functional level with minimal risk and problems by the time of discharge. If the patient can't recover completely, your care should help him to cope physically and emotionally with his impaired or declining health.

Keeping it real

With these long-range goals in mind, you need to identify realistic, measurable expected outcomes and corresponding target dates for your patient. Expected outcomes are goals the patient should reach as a result of planned nursing interventions. Sometimes, a nursing diagnosis requires more than one expected outcome.

Outcomes are always geared toward the patient's performance—not the nurse's actions. An outcome can specify an improvement in the patient's ability to function—for example, an increase in the distance he can walk—or it can specify the correction of a problem such as a reduction in pain. In either case, each outcome calls for the maximum realistic improvement for a particular patient.

Make sure that the outcomes in your nursing care plan focus on the patient—not on actions you must perform.

The outcome statement

All outcomes must be patient oriented and expressed in the form of a statement, called the *outcome statement*. For instance, a patient with a nursing diagnosis of *Impaired gas exchange related to ventilation perfusion imbalance from pulmonary embolus* might have an expected outcome of "Show decreased work of breathing and restlessness and increased oxygen saturation within 24 hours of heparin infusion initiation."

Parts of an outcome statement

An outcome statement consists of four components:
1. a specific behavior that shows the patient has reached his goal
2. criteria for measuring that behavior
3. the conditions under which the behavior should occur
4. a time frame for when the behavior should occur. (See *Understanding outcome statements,* page 87.)

Behavior

A *behavior* is generally defined as an action that can be observed or heard. In terms of outcome identification, it is an action that you would expect to see in the patient as a result of your nursing interventions.

Objectively speaking

Always begin your outcome statement with an action verb that focuses on a behavior you can objectively observe and measure. Examples of verbs that can be easily measured by sight or sound include:
* movements (e.g., *ambulate, bathe, climb, give, move, perform, point, use*)
* speech (e.g., *describe, express, report, state, verbalize*)
* other actions (e.g., *arrange, avoid, demonstrate, exhibit, identify, maintain, modify, participate, seek, set*).

Sounds subjective to me

Although it's important to consider the patient's thoughts and feelings when planning care, these can't be readily observed or measured. Avoid beginning an outcome statement with a verb that's too subjective to evaluate, such as *accept, know, appreciate,* or *understand.* After all, how can you objectively observe a patient's *appreciation?* Even when working with a psychiatric patient, you'll write outcomes based on behaviors—not the thoughts or feelings that might be influencing the behaviors. For example, instead of including the outcome "Patient will state that he feels less depressed," you might include the outcome "Patient will obtain a score of less than 10 on the Beck Depression Scale"; this outcome is a measurable improvement in a patient's mood.

Measure

Explaining precisely what's being measured and how it's being measured helps gauge your patient's progress toward

Memory jogger

To remember the four necessary components of an effective outcome statement, think, "**B**e **M**ore **C**areful, **T**immy":

BMCT

Behavior

Measure

Conditions

Time frame.

I object to subjective outcome statements. Make sure that your nursing outcomes focus on behaviors that can be objectively observed or measured.

Understanding outcome statements

An outcome statement consists of four elements: behavior, measure, condition, and time frame.

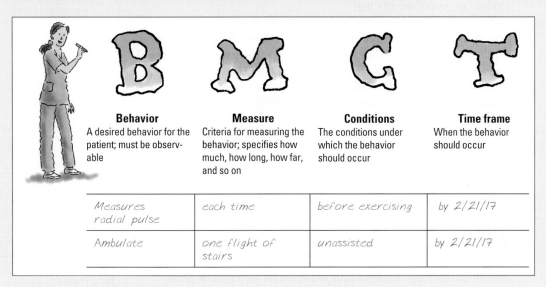

	Behavior	Measure	Conditions	Time frame
	A desired behavior for the patient; must be observable	Criteria for measuring the behavior; specifies how much, how long, how far, and so on	The conditions under which the behavior should occur	When the behavior should occur
	Measures radial pulse	each time	before exercising	by 2/21/17
	Ambulate	one flight of stairs	unassisted	by 2/21/17

achieving his goal. It also enables you and other team members to work within consistent parameters, ensuring the systematic evaluation of nursing interventions.

Specifics, please

Make sure your outcome statement indicates the criteria needed to measure the behavior, such as:

- how much
- how long
- how far
- using what scale.

Conditions

Stipulate in the outcome statement, as necessary, the conditions under which the behavior should occur. For instance, tell when during the day the behavior should occur, how frequently it should occur, and whether the patient requires any assistance in completing the action.

For example, the outcome statement, "Patient will drink 360 mL of noncaffeinated fluids on day shift, 240 mL on evening shift, and 120 mL on night shift," gives more direction to staff and sets a clearer goal for the patient than the statement "Patient will drink 720 mL of noncaffeinated fluids per day."

Memory jogger

To differentiate objective from subjective patient behavior, think in terms of what you need to do to interpret it:

Objective—Observe directly through sight or sound.

Subjective—Sense what the patient is thinking or feeling.

Don't set the bar too high

Keep in mind your patient's overall condition, ability to perform the behavior, and agreement with the proposed target. Make sure the conditions can be realistically met.

For example, you're caring for a patient who has had an acute exacerbation of moderate chronic obstructive lung disease and now requires oxygen therapy for exertion and sleep. The patient's nursing diagnoses include *Deficient knowledge related to misconceptions about COPD and oxygen therapy as evidenced by verbal statements regarding the disease* and *Activity intolerance related to COPD as evidenced by exertional dyspnea.* You're aware that mild but regular exercise, such as performing self-bathing and grooming activities, can help the patient maintain his residual pulmonary function, so you establish an expected outcome of "Bathe independently except for back and lower legs daily within 2 weeks." However, this outcome may not be realistic unless the patient responds to your teaching plan for *Deficient knowledge.* If the patient doesn't understand the basis for your outcome statement or doesn't agree that the goal is achievable, the expected outcome isn't realistic. In this situation, your outcome timing for the *Deficient knowledge* diagnosis must be set before the target date on the bathing outcome, and you must be prepared to adjust the bathing outcome statement depending on the patient's response to the teaching plan.

Keep time in mind. Remember to include a time frame for completing each outcome.

Time frame

Although one of your primary responsibilities as a nurse is to help your patient achieve the highest level of functioning before discharge, you need some way of monitoring his progress along the way. All patient outcomes must provide a *realistic time frame* for completing the *desired behavior.* For example, in a student care plan for a home care patient you'll be seeing once a week, you might have a new outcome statement for each visit, as you assist the patient to learn to manage his disease process. At some point in his care, you may then be able to write a longer outcome target as he gradually integrates new information and techniques into his daily routine.

The long and short of goals

Long-term goals commonly require weeks or months to achieve. Short-term goals, on the other hand, take much less time to achieve; these are typically the goals (or outcomes) you'll address in your outcome statement. (See *Documenting long-term goals.*)

Documenting long-term goals

As a student, the expected outcomes of the patient that you write will generally reflect short-term goals. Your instructors focus your care plans on patient outcomes that are achievable by you during your limited clinical time with a specific patient. However, to demonstrate that you're aware of the larger issues involved in caring for a patient, you'll also probably be asked to document discharge planning. This is where you'll express the patient's long-term goals. Some of the items you may be asked to include are:

• discharge outcomes—specify the outcomes expected by the time of discharge

• learning needs—list the topics that the patient and family should demonstrate an understanding of by discharge

• referrals—explain possible referrals needed to assist the patient and his family in reaching long-term optimum health outcomes

• documentation issues—identify the results of outcome evaluation that must be documented.

To each his own

As a practicing nurse, your agency or facility may have a different system of handling short-term and long-term outcomes in its care plans. Some examples are listed here:

• Acute-care settings: Factors affecting discharge planning are documented on the initial assessment. The nursing care plan lists outcomes expected by discharge. Teaching flow sheets and discharge instruction sheets are used to document learning need outcomes and patient status and medical orders plus any referrals or follow-up care on discharge. Patients are given a copy of their discharge instructions.

• Rehabilitative, home care, long-term-care settings: The nursing or interprofessional care plan lists short-term and long-term patient goals for each diagnosis and specifies dates for re-evaluation of each. Discharge planning begins when the patient has been appropriately re-evaluated or requests discharge. Preparations for discharge are then listed as a patient goal on the updated care plan, as are any continuing patient care needs and referrals. A discharge summary is completed on the day of discharge and a copy is given to the patient.

Find out and follow the documentation procedures at your facility.

Writing outcome statements

When writing outcome statements, always start with a *specific action verb* that focuses on your patient's behavior. By telling how your patient should look, walk, eat, turn, cough, speak, or stand, for example, you give a clear picture of how to evaluate progress.

Choose wisely

Be careful about your verb choice, though. Such verbs as "allow," "let," and "enable" focus attention on your own and other health care team member's behavior—not the patient's behavior. In many cases, you can easily turn around outcome statements that focus on your behavior so that they focus on the patient. For example, "Medication brings chest pain relief" doesn't say anything about the patient's behavior, but "Expresses relief from chest pain within 5 minutes of receiving medication" does.

Teacher knows best

Tips for keeping statements concise

These tips will help you write clear, precise patient outcome statements:

• **Avoid unnecessary words.** For example, with many documentation formats, you won't need to include the phrase "The patient will…" with each expected outcome statement. In most cases, it's obvious that you're talking about the patient. However, you'll have to specify which person the goals refer to when family, friends, or others are involved.

• **Use accepted abbreviations.** Refer to The Joint Commission's and your facility's list of approved abbreviations. If your facility's list describes patient stays in day-long intervals, use abbreviations such as "HD1" for hospital day 1 or "POD 2" for postoperative day 2.

• **Use a standardized list of patient outcomes,** such as the Nursing Outcomes Classification or the classification system used in your facility.

Include the nitty-gritty

Also be sure to make your statements specific. For example, the statement "Understands relaxation techniques" doesn't tell you much. (How do you observe a patient's understanding?) Instead, you should write: "Practices progressive muscle relaxation techniques unassisted for 15 minutes daily by hospital day 5." This statement tells you exactly what to look for when assessing the patient's progress. Choose your words carefully and be clear and concise. (See *Tips for keeping statements concise,* above.)

For your consideration

When writing outcome statements, consider the patient's medical orders. The outcome statements you write shouldn't ignore or contradict those medical orders. For example, before including the outcome statement, "Ambulate 10′ unassisted twice per day by postoperative day 3," make sure that the medical orders don't call for more restricted activity.

Also, adapt the outcome to the specific circumstances. Consider such health-related factors as the patient's coping ability, age, education, cultural influences, family support, living conditions, socioeconomic status, and anticipated length of stay. Also consider the health care setting. For example, the outcome statement, "Ambulate outdoors with assistance for 20 minutes t.i.d. by admission day 5," might be unrealistic in a facility located within a large city. (See *Factors affecting health.*)

Although your outcome statements should be detailed, try to keep them clear and concise.

Factors affecting health

Various factors can affect your patient's overall health and ability to achieve wellness. Keep these factors in mind when developing or modifying a patient care plan.

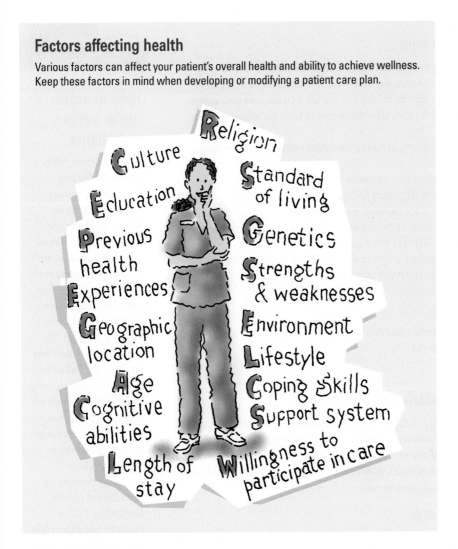

Culture
Religion
Education
Standard of living
Previous health Experiences
Genetics
Strengths & weaknesses
Geographic location
Environment
Lifestyle
Age
Coping Skills
Cognitive abilities
Support system
Length of stay
Willingness to participate in care

Patient participation

One way to help ensure the effectiveness of outcome statements is to encourage the patient to participate in formulating them. A patient who helps write his outcome statements is more motivated to achieve his goals. His input, along with family member input, can also help you set realistic goals. (See *Eliciting the patient's help* and *How to obtain better patient compliance,* page 92.)

Up for a challenge?

Not all outcome statements will be as straightforward to formulate as the examples previously presented. In such cases, remembering the four components and identifying each component separately can help

Eliciting the patient's help

Discussing the care plan with patients and keeping them informed about their progress and needed changes can be mutually beneficial. The patient remains informed and actively involved in health care decisions, and you elicit compliance with achieving the outcomes stipulated in the care plan. Remember to keep the following points in mind:

• Discuss the care plan with patients, and keep them informed whenever the plan changes.
• Assess patient knowledge about their condition or problem.
• Explain procedures and review laboratory findings.
• Respect the patient's wishes in the decision-making process.
• Begin discussing discharge plans at the earliest appropriate time, keeping the patient apprised of necessary changes to the plan.
• Seek patient permission to discuss progress and needs with family members or significant others, particularly when planning ahead toward discharge.

Weighing the evidence

How to obtain better patient compliance

In a 2004 article in the *Journal of Nursing Care Quality*, authors Maramba, Richards, Myers, and Larrabee reported their literature review research on the discharge planning process. One of the components investigated was patient satisfaction with the care provided. The authors stated that "Two studies identified patient and family understanding of the patient's condition, feeling prepared to manage care after discharge, and being involved in decisions related to discharge planning as predictors of patient satisfaction." Other research has shown that when patients are more satisfied with their care, they're more likely to follow the care plan on discharge.

you formulate outcome statements. (See *Finding the right words in difficult situations,* pages 93–94.)

Nursing Outcomes Classification

As described in Chapter 1, the Nursing Outcomes Classification (NOC) is a nursing-sensitive, standardized categorization of patient outcomes that helps nurses evaluate the effects of nursing interventions. Experience has shown, however, that the outcomes listed can be useful for other disciplines as well.

Just so we understand each other...

In order to correlate patient outcomes with specific interventions and evaluate their effectiveness in a way that's meaningful and useful, health care providers must agree on standardized definitions of the words used when talking about patient care. Such standardization serves four main purposes:

• It ensures consistent measurement and comparison of patient outcomes.
• It helps validate the effectiveness of nursing care as a component of quality, cost-effective health care.
• It further legitimizes the profession of nursing in the health care arena.
• It aids in adapting nursing care planning into the electronic health system database.

(*Text continues on page 94.*)

Finding the right words in difficult situations

Some of the most difficult nursing diagnoses to work with are those that reflect the patient's perceptions and feelings and those that refer to normal human processes such as birth. Let's look at and work through two examples.

Example diagnosis 1

In some ways, the diagnosis *Risk for disorganized infant behavior related to potential intrapartum complications* appears to have a simple outcome: the fetus will be delivered without experiencing any alteration in normal fetal signs indicative of intrapartum complications resulting in disorganized infant behavior. But how do you word the behavior, measure, condition, and time frame in the outcome statement for this generalized outcome?

One step at a time

Here are four steps for constructing an outcome statement for this diagnosis:
- Consider what actual fetal signs you can measure while the infant is in the process of being delivered (the mother is in labor). Examples might include fetal heart rate, variations in electronic fetal monitoring patterns, the presence of meconium staining of the amniotic fluid when the sac has broken, and fetal position or presenting part. Then think of an action verb to describe the **behavior** (sign) you want to see. Examples might include "Maintain fetal heart rate" or "Detect meconium staining of the amniotic fluid."
- Determine the limits for the behavior—in other words, the way in which you would **measure** the success or failure of your outcome. For "Maintain fetal heart rate," you would want to specify the normal fetal heart rate range during labor, which is 120 to 160 beats/minute. For "Detect meconium staining of amniotic fluid," you would expect the amniotic fluid to be clear or have a yellow or green tinge on rupture of the amniotic sac, not marked by the dark green color of meconium. If staining were present, the infant would be at risk for aspiration of meconium during the intrapartum period.
- Outline the **conditions** under which you would expect to find the two behaviors listed above. In normal labor, the fetal heart rate would remain within the cited limits throughout the delivery process. But detection of the color of the amniotic fluid (the indicator for the risk of aspiration of meconium) must be stated more specifically, by saying, for example, "immediately," "within 5 minutes," "within 2 hours," or whatever time you believe is realistic considering the situation.

- Last, state the **time frame** within which you would expect to accomplish the stated outcomes. In this situation, the time frame can be the period ending with the birth of the infant or, for the amniotic fluid, the time after the amniotic sac has broken.

Putting it together

For this diagnosis, you could make two clear outcome statements using the guidelines above:
- Maintain fetal heart rate within 120 to 160 beats/minute throughout the intrapartum period until birth.
- Detect meconium staining of the amniotic fluid by presence of dark green color of the fluid within 5 minutes of rupture of the amniotic sac.

As you can probably see, several other possibilities for specific outcome statements exist for this diagnosis. As a student, you would choose only those for which you could be accountable during your clinical time with the patient.

Example diagnosis 2

Let's look at another example with a different type of diagnosis: *Ineffective denial related to new diagnosis of pulmonary hypertension as evidenced by patient statements, "I feel better already. You just let me go home, and I'll get back to work in no time" and "I think I was just working too much overtime and got exhausted. I just needed a break."* The first tendency would be to write the outcome statement: "Patient will accept his new diagnosis of pulmonary hypertension by discharge." However, because "accept" is a subjective verb, this outcome is hard to measure. Taking one component at a time, let's see how to word a reasonable outcome for this patient:
- Objective desired patient **behaviors** might include "Describes pulmonary hypertension as the source of changes in functional capacity," "Expresses interest in learning more about pulmonary hypertension," "States understanding of the chronic and progressive nature of pulmonary hypertension," and "Questions staff about how pulmonary hypertension may affect his ability to return to work after hospital discharge."

The creators of NOC have done extensive research with practicing nurses and nurse-educators in various settings to determine which words nurses regularly use in discussing the outcomes of their patient care and which tasks they perform to impact these outcomes. NOC research is ongoing to validate each outcome and indicator as well as to add new outcomes.

What NOC is not

Perhaps the most confusing thing about using NOC is understanding that a NOC outcome *isn't* the same as a nursing goal or expected outcome. By definition, it's an individual patient's state or behavior, including perceptions or subjective states. In fact, NOC outcomes are deliberately designed to be variable, not goal specific. What does this mean? It means that an NOC outcome:

• defines a patient's state at a specific time, which can represent an improvement or a decline from that patient's state at an earlier assessment
• becomes an "outcome" only if it's assessed after a nursing intervention (thus, a patient's mobility status on an admission assessment is information, not an outcome)
• is measured along a continuum from negative to positive
• has an associated group of specific state, behavior, or perception descriptions (called *indicators*) that give examples of the various components of the outcome
• can apply to any discipline if it uses indicators representative of the discipline instead of the nursing indicators listed in NOC
• can be reformatted into a nursing goal (outcome statement or expected outcome) when used with its indicators and in conjunction with an expected completion date.

How the taxonomy works

NOC is a five-component classification system that's categorized according to:

• health domain
• outcome class

Don't be afraid of NOC. There are several advantages to using the standardized language that NOC offers.

- outcome labels
- indicators of the outcomes
- measures of the outcomes and indicators.

The big breakdown

Seven different domains and 31 classes are identified in NOC. The domains are:
- functional health
- physiological health
- psychosocial health
- health knowledge and behavior
- perceived health
- family health
- community health.

NOC around the clock

NOC currently includes 490 research-based outcomes, each with its own four-digit taxonomy number, standardized definition, and list of indicators (behavioral criteria by which the more general outcome can be evaluated). To assist in quantifying the behaviors listed, a five-point Likert-type scale is identified for each outcome. (See *Get to know Likert scales—Likert or not*, below.) Users of the system are encouraged, though not mandated, to use the scales provided in order to maintain reliability and validity of outcome measurement. The system also provides a space for the nurse to

Get to know Likert scales—Likert or not

A Likert scale, named after Rensis Likert, is a type of psychometric response scale commonly used in questionnaires. Traditionally, this scale has been used to gauge a participant's level of agreement with a particular statement. For example, a participant might be asked to rate his level of agreement with the statement, "I like ice cream," using a five-point scale that includes "Strongly agree," "Agree," "Neither agree nor disagree," "Disagree," and "Strongly disagree." Each of the categories is assigned a number (e.g., "Strongly agree" = 4; "Agree" = 3; "Neither agree nor disagree" = 2, "Disagree" = 1; and "Strongly disagree" = 0) that allows the scale to be scored. Scores for several items are usually combined to provide an overall rating. Likert scales can have more or less than five points; however, five are commonly used. If Likert scales seem familiar to you, you might have encountered them on a course evaluation form.

Ice cream? I strongly agree!

document an outcome target rating for the patient. (See *Anatomy of a NOC outcome,* page 97.)

Practice your scales

The Likert scales in the NOC system allow nurses (and other members of the health care team) to evaluate the patient's status from most negative to most positive over time. Examples of scales commonly used to track outcomes include:

Extremely compromised 1	Substantially compromised 2	Moderately compromised 3	Mildly compromised 4	Not compromised 5

Never demonstrated 1	Rarely demonstrated 2	Sometimes demonstrated 3	Often demonstrated 4	Consistently demonstrated 5

None 1	Limited 2	Moderate 3	Substantial 4	Extensive 5

Using NOC to write expected outcomes

Although NOC outcomes aren't the same as expected outcomes, you can use NOC to write outcome statements. Here's how:
- Go to the "NANDA International–NOC Linkages" section of the NOC text and find each of the nursing diagnoses you've selected for your patient. Below each one, you'll see the NANDA International (NANDA-I) definition of the diagnosis and then lists of suggested outcomes and associated outcomes. (See *Speaking the language,* page 98.)
- Choose outcomes from the lists that seem like they might apply to your patient.
- Find each of the potential outcomes in the alphabetical listing in the NOC text, and read the outcome definition and indicators to determine whether the outcome is appropriate for your patient.
- For each appropriate outcome, choose the indicators that apply to your patient.
- Assign baseline ratings for each indicator as well as an overall baseline rating.
- Allocate an overall target rating for the patient and a time frame for achieving the goal based on the patient's assessment data, current condition, and personal goals. (See *NOC outcomes.*)

Anatomy of a NOC outcome

Becoming familiar with the organization and components of an individual NOC outcome can help you to use NOC to write specific outcome statements for your patients. Below is a sample outcome.

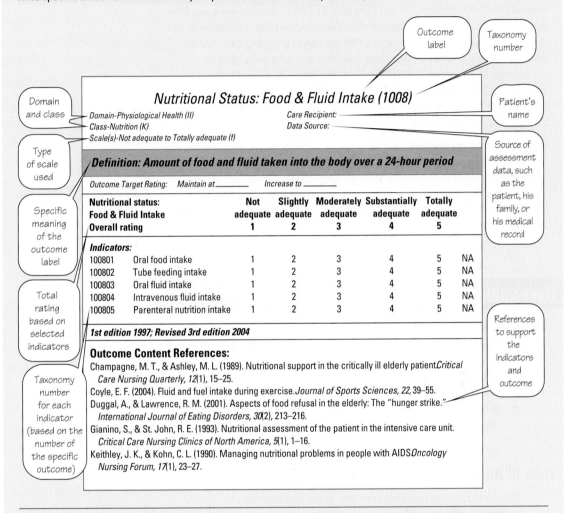

Used from Moorhead, S., et al. (2013). *Nursing outcomes classification (NOC)* (5th ed.). St. Louis, MO: Mosby, with permission.

Speaking the language

Once you start working with the Nursing Outcomes Classification (NOC), you'll quickly realize that the NOC domains are different from the domains listed in NANDA International (NANDA-I) taxonomy. As you'll see later on, both of these domains also differ from the domains in the Nursing Interventions Classification (NIC). The reason for this is that each language is trying to codify a different aspect of nursing care. To successfully incorporate each of these taxonomies into your care plans, refer to:

Johnson, M, Moorhead, S, Bulechek, G. M., Butcher, H. K., Maas, M., & Swanson, E. (2012). *NOC and NIC linkages to NANDA-I and clinical conditions: Supporting critical reasoning and quality care, 3e (NANDA, NOC, and NIC linkages)* (3rd ed.). St. Louis, MO: Mosby.

Improving for the greater good

In 2000, representatives from NANDA-I, NIC, and NOC created the NNN Alliance, a virtual organization aimed at fostering a working relationship among the three organizations. One goal of this alliance has been to develop a more universal language that can be used not only for these taxonomies but also for other nursing languages.

Developing nursing interventions

Once you've developed expected outcomes for a patient, it's time to start planning specific interventions to achieve them. As with patient outcomes, nursing interventions must be:
- realistic
- measurable
- achievable within the time frame specified in the patient outcome.

Types of interventions

Interventions are grouped into two general categories:
- independent
- collaborative (or interdependent).

Independent interventions

An independent intervention is one that falls within the scope of nursing practice. It doesn't require a practitioner's (physician or nurse practitioner) direction or supervision, nurses can initiate the action on their own.

Under construction

NOC outcomes

Like all expected outcomes, the outcomes you develop based on the Nursing Outcomes Classification (NOC) should contain the following elements: behavior, measure, criteria, and time frame. However, the form these elements take is modified by the structure of the language of NOC. The examples shown here illustrate two ways in which you might record an NOC expected outcome in your care plan. The actual format you use is determined by your school or facility.

NOC format
This format records the outcome statement in the chart form given in the NOC text.

> *Fill in the patient's target goal rating here. Note that this goal can be either a maintenance goal or an improvement goal.*

> *Circle the patient's baseline ratings for the indicators that you select here.*

Nutritional Status: Food & Fluid Intake (1008)

Domain-Physiological Health (II) *Care Recipient:Susan Wong*
Class-Nutrition (K) *Data Source:Patient, chart*
Scale(s)-Not adequate to Totally adequate (f)

> *Circle the patient's overall baseline rating here.*

Definition: Amount of food and fluid taken into the body over a 24-hour period

Outcome Target Rating: Maintain at _____   Increase to 4_____   within 7 days

Nutritional status: Food & Fluid Intake	Not adequate	Slightly adequate	Moderately adequate	Substantially adequate	Totally adequate	
Overall rating	1	2	(3)	4	5	
Indicators:						
100801 Oral food intake	1	2	(3)	4	5	NA
100802 Tube feeding intake	1	2	3	4	5	(NA)
100803 Oral fluid intake	1	2	(3)	4	5	NA
100804 Intravenous fluid intake	1	2	3	4	5	(NA)
100805 Parenteral nutrition intake	1	2	3	4	5	(NA)

1st edition 1997; Revised 3rd edition 2004

> *Circle "NA" for any indicators that you haven't chosen for your patient.*

> *If a copy of the outcome is included in the medical record, sign the outcome and include the date of the assessment.*

Outcome Content References:
Champagne, M. T., & Ashley, M. L. (1989). Nutritional support in the critically ill elderly patient.*Critical Care Nursing Quarterly, 12*(1), 15–25.
Coyle, E. F. (2004). Fluid and fuel intake during exercise*Journal of Sports Sciences, 22,*39–55.
Duggal, A., & Lawrence, R. M. (2001). Aspects of food refusal in the elderly: The "hunger strike." *International Journal of Eating Disorders, 30* (2), 213–216.
Gianino, S., & St. John, R. E. (1993). Nutritional assessment of the patient in the intensive care unit. *Critical Care Nursing Clinics of North America, 5* (1), 1–16.
Keithley, J. K., & Kohn, C. L. (1990). Managing nutritional problems in people with AIDS*Oncology Nursing Forum, 17*(1), 23–27.

Joan Cunningham, RN
3/14/12

NOC outcomes (*continued*)

NOC format

This example condenses the information from NOC into a simpler format that is commonly used in schools.

Code or label	Definition and indicators	Measure	Time frame
1008	Nutritional Status: Food & Fluid Intake The amount of food and fluid taken into the body over a 24-hour period		
100801	Oral food intake	at a level of 4 (substantially adequate)	within 7 days
100803	Oral fluid intake	at a level of 4 (substantially adequate)	within 7 days

Remember that you shouldn't change the NOC outcome label and definition; however, you can add new indicators or modify existing ones to make them more specific to your patient. For example, you could redefine the measurement of indicator 100801 of the Nutritional Status: Food and Fluid Intake NOC outcome (Oral food intake) to make it more specific (for instance, by defining 1 = no intake; 2 = 25% of food available per meal; 3 = 50% of food available per meal; 4 = 75% of food available per meal; and 5 = 100% of food available per meal).

You're on your own, kid

Many of the interventions you'll incorporate into the care plan are independent nursing interventions. They address aspects of care that nurses can do to promote change and facilitate wellness. These interventions cover such topics as:
- performing activities of daily living
- promoting safety and comfort
- patient teaching.

Independent interventions involve working directly with a patient, such as teaching him how to perform his own insulin injections. However, they also include the indirect activities you pursue to help him reach his goal, such as gathering resource materials about diabetes and insulin self-injection.

Independent interventions don't require any direction or supervision from a practitioner.

Collaborative interventions

A collaborative intervention is one that's based on instructions (oral or written) provided by a practitioner (physician or nurse practitioner) or one that you'll do in consultation with another member of the health care team, such as a dietitian, social worker, or physical therapist. Collaborative interprofessional interventions fall outside the realm of nursing practice, meaning that you can't initiate them on your own.

Hey, let's work together

Examples of collaborative interprofessional interventions include:
- administering prescribed medications or fluids
- obtaining specimens for laboratory analysis
- diagnostic procedures such as imaging, X-ray
- exercise prescription by physical therapy
- nutritional assessment by the dietician.

    (See *Comparing independent and collaborative nursing interventions,* page 102.)

Collaborative interventions are ones that you perform based on the instructions from another member of the health care team.

Writing nursing interventions

All nursing interventions are based on the goals stated in the patient outcomes and are intended to alter the etiology, symptoms, or risk factors for a specific nursing diagnosis. The number of nursing interventions can vary for each outcome. What's most important is that the care plan is comprehensive enough to ensure that the patient can meet the outcomes. You'll usually list several nursing interventions covering various aspects of care, all aimed at correcting the problem identified in the nursing diagnosis.

Each nursing intervention you "prescribe" must be written so that a caregiver (nurse's assistant or another nurse) has a clear picture of what to do to promote a positive change in the patient. As a student, your care plans are generally completed for your instructor, not for the agency or facility where you gain your clinical experience. (See *Tips for writing effective nursing interventions,* page 103.)

Identify the activity

Keep in mind that all interventions are actions that *you* or another nurse or nurse's assistant (not the patient) will do. Therefore, they should always begin with an action verb, for example:
- *Offer* fluids every 4 hours.
- *Monitor* temperature, blood pressure, and pulse.
- *Assess* pedal pulses.
- *Discuss* with patient how to perform regular self-breast exams.

Comparing independent and collaborative nursing interventions

Differentiating independent nursing interventions from collaborative interprofessional interventions can be difficult. Some interventions can be classified as either independent or interdependent, depending on the wording used for the intervention and the nurse's understanding of their scope of practice. One way to differentiate is to consider whether the action is nurse prescribed or practitioner (physician or nurse practitioner) prescribed.

This chart demonstrates a chain of related independent nursing interventions and interprofessional collaborative actions related to a practitioner (physician or nurse practitioner) order for bed rest.

Tips for writing effective interventions

To write interventions clearly and correctly, follow these guidelines:

• Keep your interventions simple and to the point, and make sure they're aimed at helping your patient achieve the desired outcome.

• Clearly state the necessary action. Note how and when to perform the intervention, and include special instructions if necessary. For example, "Promote comfort" doesn't tell you what specific action to take, but "Administer ordered analgesic 30 minutes before dressing change" specifies exactly what to do and when to do it.

• Make sure your interventions fit the patient. Consider the patient's age, condition, developmental level, environment, and values. For instance, if the patient is a vegetarian, don't write an intervention that requires him to eat lean meat to gain extra pounds for healing.

• Keep the patient's safety in mind. Consider his physical and mental limitations. For instance, before teaching a patient how to self-administer medication, make sure he's physically able to do it and that he can remember and follow the regimen.

• Follow your facility's rules. For example, if your facility allows only nurses to administer medications, don't write an intervention calling for the patient to administer hemorrhoidal suppositories as needed.

• Consider other health care activities. Adjust your interventions when other activities interfere with them. For example, you might want your patient to get plenty of rest on a day when he has several diagnostic tests scheduled.

• Use available resources. If your patient needs to learn about his cardiac problem, use your facility's education department, literature from the American Heart Association, and local support groups. Write your intervention to reflect the use of these resources.

• Unlike outcomes, which are patient focused, interventions focus on the actions that you, the nurse, will take.

Make it specific

Include as many specific qualifiers as possible:
• how, when, and where to do the activity
• how frequently it needs to be done
• special equipment needed
• additional instructions.

Watch the time

Remember that all of the interventions developed for a particular patient outcome must be achievable within the same time frame.

This doesn't mean, however, that a particular intervention can't be used again to meet a new progressive outcome related to the original diagnosis.

Keep in mind

When planning interventions, give some thought to:
- likelihood of success, taking into account the timing, interventions by other team members, amount of time required, and cost factors
- resources available to you and your patient
- the ability to perform the intervention
- scientific rationale behind the actions
- the patient's ability and willingness to comply
- prior interventions that you or your patient have successfully used
- interventions from standardized care plans, nursing textbooks, or nursing journals. (See *Plan to succeed.*)

Unlike outcomes, which are patient focused, interventions focus on the actions that you, the nurse, will take.

Nursing Interventions Classification

The Nursing Interventions Classification (NIC) is a systematized classification of research-based nursing interventions. NIC interventions cover such areas as illness prevention, illness treatment, and health promotion. Most are designed for individual patients, but some are geared toward families and communities. Covering a broad range of nursing care, NIC may be used in any practice setting and any specialty across the entire health care continuum—from intensive care to primary care, home care, and hospice. Like NOC, NIC is designed so that even non–nurse health care providers can use the interventions in their treatment of patients. The most difficult aspect of using NIC for nurses new to the language is that instead of listing the specific actions the nurse will take, NIC uses labels that group several actions (called *activities*) together.

Class act

NIC consists of 554 interventions (both physiological and psychosocial labels) that are grouped into 30 classes and 7 domains. The 7 domains are unique to NIC and don't correlate directly with the NANDA-I or NOC domains. They are:
- physiological (basic)—supports physical functioning
- physiological (complex)—supports homeostatic regulation
- behavioral—supports social function and lifestyle changes
- safety—supports protection against harm

Plan to succeed

Always consider your intervention options carefully, and then weigh their potential for success. Determine if you can obtain the necessary equipment and resources. If not, take steps to get what you need or change the intervention accordingly. Also, observe the patient's willingness and functional ability to participate in the various interventions, and be prepared to postpone or modify them if necessary. For example, don't plan extensive verbal teaching with a patient who has significant hearing loss.

- family—supports the family unit
- health system—supports use of the health care system
- community—supports health of the community.

    Each intervention in the classification includes a taxonomic code, a label name, a definition, and a list of activities to carry out the intervention. Nurses can select specific activities based on patient need and circumstances. (See *Anatomy of a NIC intervention,* page 106.)

Using NIC to write interventions

Just as you may be asked to use NOC to create your expected outcome statements, you may be asked to choose interventions from a standardized interventions classification, such as NIC. You can find the information in the *Nursing Interventions Classification* book in two ways. First, you can look in the alphabetical listing for the intervention you're interested in. If you find the list daunting or you've looked up what you believe to be key words or concepts for an intervention and haven't found what you wanted, you can search for interventions using NANDA-I nursing diagnoses. *Nursing Interventions Classification* includes charts that list NANDA-I nursing diagnoses alphabetically, with the diagnosis definition and suggested and optional nursing interventions for each diagnosis.

Personalization

Remember that NIC includes a definition for each class of interventions that shouldn't be changed. However, NIC is designed to be dynamic and flexible, allowing nurses to modify the activities to reflect the unique needs of the patient and his family. Interventions from more than one class may be needed to help the patient achieve his expected outcomes. Nurses can also add activities as appropriate for the patient's particular situation. (See *Getting the knack of NIC.*)

Anatomy of a NIC intervention

Becoming familiar with the organization and components of an individual Nursing Interventions Classification (NIC) can help you to use NIC to write nursing interventions specific to your patients. Below is a sample intervention and its corresponding activities.

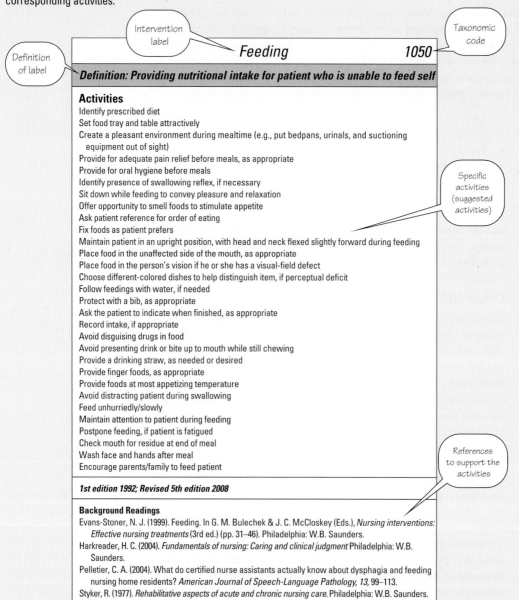

Intervention label

Taxonomic code

Definition of label

Feeding   1050

Definition: Providing nutritional intake for patient who is unable to feed self

Activities
Identify prescribed diet
Set food tray and table attractively
Create a pleasant environment during mealtime (e.g., put bedpans, urinals, and suctioning
    equipment out of sight)
Provide for adequate pain relief before meals, as appropriate
Provide for oral hygiene before meals
Identify presence of swallowing reflex, if necessary
Sit down while feeding to convey pleasure and relaxation
Offer opportunity to smell foods to stimulate appetite
Ask patient reference for order of eating
Fix foods as patient prefers
Maintain patient in an upright position, with head and neck flexed slightly forward during feeding
Place food in the unaffected side of the mouth, as appropriate
Place food in the person's vision if he or she has a visual-field defect
Choose different-colored dishes to help distinguish item, if perceptual deficit
Follow feedings with water, if needed
Protect with a bib, as appropriate
Ask the patient to indicate when finished, as appropriate
Record intake, if appropriate
Avoid disguising drugs in food
Avoid presenting drink or bite up to mouth while still chewing
Provide a drinking straw, as needed or desired
Provide finger foods, as appropriate
Provide foods at most appetizing temperature
Avoid distracting patient during swallowing
Feed unhurriedly/slowly
Maintain attention to patient during feeding
Postpone feeding, if patient is fatigued
Check mouth for residue at end of meal
Wash face and hands after meal
Encourage parents/family to feed patient

Specific activities (suggested activities)

References to support the activities

1st edition 1992; Revised 5th edition 2008

Background Readings
Evans-Stoner, N. J. (1999). Feeding. In G. M. Bulechek & J. C. McCloskey (Eds.), *Nursing interventions:
    Effective nursing treatments* (3rd ed.) (pp. 31–46). Philadelphia: W.B. Saunders.
Harkreader, H. C. (2004). *Fundamentals of nursing: Caring and clinical judgment* Philadelphia: W.B.
    Saunders.
Pelletier, C. A. (2004). What do certified nurse assistants actually know about dysphagia and feeding
    nursing home residents? *American Journal of Speech-Language Pathology, 13,* 99–113.
Styker, R. (1977). *Rehabilitative aspects of acute and chronic nursing care.* Philadelphia: W.B. Saunders.

Using evidence–based practice

Evidence-based practice can be defined as the systematic and judicious use of the current best evidence to make decisions about patient care. When applied to nursing, the term *evidence-based practice* is used to describe the care that nurses provide based on research and identified standards.

Shifting sands

Because of the vast amount of available clinical research and accessibility to research findings, there has been a steady shift away from traditional, intuitive-oriented nursing toward evidence-based nursing. Nurses are following the growing trend among all health care fields of using well-designed and well-executed scientific studies to guide their clinical decision-making and clinical care.

Putting evidence into practice

For your student care plans, your instructor may require you to write scientific, evidence-based rationales for the nursing interventions you've planned or completed. Students are also required to provide a complete reference list regarding their scientific rationales. Evidence-based, scientific rationales can come from textbooks, peer-reviewed journal articles, or reputable internet Web sites. Be careful about citing from Internet-based Web sites—not all information on the Internet is accurate.

When planning care, you should use evidence-based research and your critical thinking skills to ascertain why certain actions or practices are being performed. Asking pertinent questions can help you determine whether you're taking the right course of action and whether the interventions you've chosen will improve your patient's outcome.

Although tradition has its time and place, evidence-based practice ensures that nurses keep up with the times by using clinically sound best practices.

Don't be afraid to ask

Questions to ask yourself as you plan nursing interventions include the following:
- Who determined the basis for this treatment?
- Is there a scientific rationale for the treatment or practice?
- What's the rationale for this treatment or practice in relation to this patient?
- What are the clinical consequences and potential complications of this practice?
- Is this the only way of performing this procedure?
- Could this treatment be performed more safely, more efficiently, or more cost-effectively?

Getting the knack of NIC

To better understand NIC, consider this example: You're caring for an elderly man who has Alzheimer's disease. The patient needs assistance with feeding but has no difficulty swallowing.

Using NIC

To determine interventions for this patient using NIC, take a step-by-step approach:
• Determine that the Nursing Outcomes Classification (NOC) entry *Nutritional Status: Food & Fluid Intake* is appropriate for your patient and use this NOC outcome to set outcome goals.
• Look up the corresponding NANDA International diagnosis, *Self-care deficit: Feeding*, in the *Nursing Interventions Classification* book.
• Read through each of the suggested NIC classes that might apply to your patient and choose activities that most closely represent the actions you would need to take, based on your knowledge and research. For example:
  ○ environmental management
  ○ feeding
  ○ nutrition management
  ○ nutritional monitoring
  ○ positioning.
  Note: "Bottle feeding" isn't relevant for your patient because he's an adult and "Swallowing therapy" isn't relevant to your patient because he isn't having difficulty swallowing.
• Modify or add to the listed activities as needed. For example:
  ○ Of the 30 activities, you eliminate seven as not being applicable to your patient.
  ○ You modify "Protect with a bib, as appropriate" to read "Protect with a cloth napkin" because you know the patient's spouse has brought napkins and this activity conserves the patient's self-esteem.
  ○ You modify "Record intake, if appropriate" to read "Record fluid intake on I&O sheet; record percentage of food eaten for each meal as 25%, 50%, 75%, or 100%."
  ○ You add interventions to "Weigh patient weekly," "Monitor trends in weight loss and gain," "Monitor albumin, total protein, and hemoglobin levels and hematocrit as ordered," and "Consult dietitian if patient doesn't respond to interventions by target date."

• Is it within the scope of nurse practice to perform the procedure or treatment?
• If delegating the task, is it within the scope of a nurse assistant's practice to perform the procedure or treatment?
• Is this the highest achievable outcome for the patient?

Evaluating sources of information

Truly evaluating the reliability and validity of the findings of a research study requires knowledge of statistics and research principles. However, keeping the following basic principles in mind can help you to identify valid sources of information that can be used to support evidence-based care—and avoid those that don't:

- Check medical resources for guidelines or standards of clinical practice related to your patient's medical diagnosis or the procedures or treatments he may be undergoing.
- Use resources written within the past 3 to 5 years, depending on your faculty's preference.
- Use reputable, well-known journals, Internet sites, and textbooks.
- Be wary of research that utilizes small sample sizes because the conclusions from this research may be too narrow to generalize to a larger population.

On the case

Case study background

You're caring for Johanna Keller, a patient with Parkinson's disease. After a recent medication adjustment, the patient's symptoms include mild, bilateral upper extremity tremors that improve with use of the arms and slowed ability to initiate and sustain gross motor movements (such as rising from a bed or chair and walking). The patient is highly motivated to remain as active as possible for as long as possible. Based on her assessment data, you establish the following nursing diagnosis: *Impaired physical mobility related to Parkinson's disease as evidenced by upper extremity tremors and decreased ability to initiate and sustain gross motor movements.*

Critical thinking exercise

1. Based on the definition in the NOC text, you determine that NOC outcome 0208 Mobility is appropriate for your patient. Use this NOC outcome statement for this patient.

Mobility (0208)

Domain—*Functional Health (I)*   Care Recipient:
Class—*Mobility (C)*   Data Source:
Scale(s)—*Severely compromised to Not compromised (a)*

Definition: Ability to move purposefully in own environment independently with or without assistive device

Outcome Target Rating: Maintain at _____   Increase to _____

Mobility Overall Rating	Severely compromised 1	Substantially compromised 2	Moderately compromised 3	Mildly compromised 4	Not compromised 5	
Indicators:						
020801 Balance	1	2	3	4	5	NA
020809 Coordination	1	2	3	4	5	NA
020810 Gait	1	2	3	4	5	NA
020803 Muscle movement	1	2	3	4	5	NA
020804 Joint movement	1	2	3	4	5	NA
020802 Body positioning performance	1	2	3	4	5	NA
020805 Transfer performance	1	2	3	4	5	NA
020811 Running	1	2	3	4	5	NA
020812 Jumping	1	2	3	4	5	NA
020813 Crawling	1	2	3	4	5	NA
020806 Walking	1	2	3	4	5	NA
020814 Moves with ease	1	2	3	4	5	NA

1st edition 1997; Revised 3rd edition 2004, Revised 5th edition, 2013.

Outcome Content References:

Maas, M. L., & Specht, J. P. (2001). Impaired physical mobility. In M. Maas, K. Buckwalter, M. Hardy, T. Tripp-Reimer, M. Titler, & J. Specht (Eds.), *Nursing care of older adults: Diagnoses, outcomes & interventions* (pp. 337–365). St. Louis, MO: Mosby.

Podsiadlo, D., & Richardson, S. (1991). The timed "Up & Go": A test of basic functional mobility for frail elderly persons. *Journal of American Geriatrics Society, 39*(2), 142–148.

Rukenstein, L. Z., Wieland, D., & Bernakei, R. (Eds.) (1995). *Geriatric assessment technology: The state of the art.* New York: Springer.

Used from Moorhead, S., et al. (2008). *Nursing outcomes classification (NOC)* (4th ed.), St. Louis, MO: Mosby, with permission.

2. Now review NIC intervention 0226, Exercise Therapy: Muscle Control. Nursing Interventions Classifications (NIC) (6th ed.), St Louis, MO: Mosby. Select at least five nursing activities from this NIC intervention that would be appropriate for this patient.

1. _____

2. _____

3. _____

4. _____

5. _____

Exercise Therapy: Muscle Control   0226

Definition: Use of specific activity or exercise protocols to enhance or restore controlled body movement

Activities

Determine patient's readiness to engage in activity or exercise protocol.

Collaborate with physical, occupational, and recreational therapists in developing and executing exercise program, as appropriate.

Consult physical therapy to determine optimal position for patient during exercise and number of repetitions for each movement pattern.

Evaluate sensory functions (e.g., vision, hearing, and proprioception).

Explain rationale for type of exercise and protocol to patient/family.

Provide patient privacy for exercising, if desired.

Adjust lighting, room temperature, and noise level to enhance patient's ability to concentrate on the exercise activity.

Sequence daily care activities to enhance effects of specific exercise therapy.

Initiate pain control measures before beginning exercise/activity.

Dress patient in nonrestrictive clothing.

Assist to maintain trunk and/or proximal joint stability during motor activity.

Apply splints to achieve stability of proximal joints involved with fine motor skills, as prescribed.

Re-evaluate need for assistive devices at regular intervals in collaboration with PT, OT, or RT.

Assist to sitting/standing position for exercise protocol, as appropriate.

Reinforce instructions provided to patient about the proper way to perform exercises to minimize injury and maximize effectiveness.

Determine accuracy of body image.

Reorient patient to body awareness.

Reorient patient to movement functions of the body.

Coach patient to visually scan affected side of body when performing ADLs or exercises, if indicated.

Provide step-by-step cueing for each motor activity during exercise or ADLs.

Instruct patient to "recite" each movement as it is being performed.

Use visual aids to facilitate learning how to perform ADLs or exercise movements, as appropriate.

Provide restful environment for patient after periods of exercise.

Assist patient to develop exercise protocol for strength, endurance, and flexibility.

Assist patient to formulate realistic, measurable goals.

(*continued*)

Use motor activities that require attention to and use of both sides of the body.

Incorporate ADLs into exercise protocol, if appropriate.

Encourage patient to practice exercises independently, as indicated.

Assist patient with/encourage patient to use warm-up and cool-down activities before and after exercise protocol.

Use tactile (and/or tapping) stimuli to minimize muscle spasm.

Assist patient to prepare and maintain a progress graph/chart to motivate adherence to exercise protocol.

Monitor patient's emotional, cardiovascular, and functional responses to exercise protocol.

Monitor patient's self-exercise for correct performance.

Evaluate patient's progress toward enhancement/restoration of body movement and function.

Provide positive reinforcement for patient's efforts in exercise and physical activity.

Collaborate with home caregivers regarding exercise protocol and ADLs.

Assist patient/caregiver to make prescribed revisions in home exercise plan, as indicated.

1st edition 1992; Revised 3rd edition 2000, Revised 6th edition, 2013.

Background Readings

Donohue, K., Miller, C., & Craig, B. (1988). Chronic alterations in mobility. In P. H. Mitchell (Ed.), *AANN's neuroscience nursing: Phenomena and practice* (pp. 319–343). Norwalk, CT: Appleton & Lange.

Glick, O. J. (1992). Interventions related to activity and movement. In G. M. Bulechek, & J. C. McCloskey (Eds.), Symposium on nursing interventions. *Nursing Clinics of North America, 27*(2), 541–568.

Hickey, J. (1992). *The clinical practice of neurological and neurosurgical nursing* (3rd ed.). Philadelphia, PA: J.B. Lippincott.

Hogue, C. (1985). Mobility. In E. G. Schneider (Ed.), *The teaching nursing home*. New York: Raven Press.

Lewis, C. B. (1989). *Improving mobility in older persons*. Rockville, MD: Aspen.

Lubkin, I. (1990). *Chronic illness: Impact and intervention* (2nd ed.). Boston, MA: Jones & Bartlett.

McFarland, G. K., & McFarlane, E. A. (1997). *Nursing diagnosis and intervention* (3rd ed.). St. Louis, MO: Mosby.

Moorhouse, M., Geissler, A., & Doenges, M. (1987). *Critical care plans, guidelines for patient care*. Philadelphia, PA: F.A. Davis.

Pender, N. J. (1987). *Health promotion nursing practice* (2nd ed.). Norwalk, CT: Appleton & Lange.

Sullivan, P., & Markos, P. (1993). *Clinical procedures in therapeutic exercise*. Norwalk, CT: Appleton & Lange.

Vogt, G., Miller, M., & Esluer, M. (1985). *Mosby's manual of neurological care*. St. Louis, MO: Mosby.

Out or in?

Read each statement. On the blank line provided, write "O" if the statement is a patient outcome or write "I" if it's a nursing intervention.

_____ 1. Assist with ambulation, as needed.

_____ 2. Demonstrate proper use of ambulation with quad cane within 4 days of discharge.

_____ 3. Administer oral analgesics three times per day, as prescribed.

_____ 4. Monitor vital signs every 4 hours until stable.

_____ 5. Offer sips of water and ice chips, as tolerated, followed by soft diet by HD 2 post-op.

_____ 6. Maintain acceptable body weight throughout length of stay.

_____ 7. Provide environmental cues (clock, calendar, pictures) to assist with orientation.

_____ 8. Encourage participation in daily self-care.

_____ 9. Avoid straining when having a bowel movement throughout hospitalization.

_____ 10. Verbalize decreased pain as evidenced by lower score on pain-rating scale within 1 week.

Answer key

Critical thinking exercise

1. The NOC outcome statement for this patient might look like this:

Mobility (0208)

Domain-Functional Health (I)
Class-Mobility (C)
Scale(s)-Not adequate to Not compromised (a)

Care Recipient: *Johanna Keller*
Data Source: *Patient, chart*

Definition: Ability to move purposefully in own environment independently with or without assistive device

Outcome Target Rating: Maintain at _____   Increase to _4_   *within 3 days*

Mobility Overall Rating	Severely compromised 1	Substantially compromised 2	Moderately compromised 3	Mildly compromised 4	Not compromised 5	
Indicators:						
020801 Balance	1	2	3	4	5	(NA)
020809 Coordination	1	2	3	(4)	5	NA
020810 Gait	1	2	3	(4)	5	NA
020803 Muscle movement	1	2	3	(4)	5	NA
020804 Joint movement	1	2	3	4	5	(NA)
020802 Body positioning performance	1	2	3	4	5	(NA)
020805 Transfer performance	1	2	3	(4)	5	NA
020811 Running	1	2	3	4	5	(NA)
020812 Jumping	1	2	3	4	5	(NA)
020813 Crawling	1	2	3	4	5	(NA)
020806 Walking	1	2	3	(4)	5	NA
020814 Moves with ease	1	2	3	4	5	(NA)

1st edition 1997; Revised 3rd edition 2004

Outcome Content References:

Maas, M. L., & Specht, J. P. (2001). Impaired physical mobility. In M. Maas, K. Buckwalter, M. Hardy, T. Tripp-Reimer, M. Titler, & J. Specht (Eds.), *Nursing care of older adults: Diagnoses, outcomes & interventions* (pp. 337-365). St. Louis: Mosby.

Podsiadlo, D., & Richardson, S. (1991). The timed "Up & Go": A test of basic functional mobility for frail elderly persons. *Journal of American Geriatrics Society, 39*(2), 142-148.

Rukenstein, L. Z., Wieland, D., & Bernakei, R. (Eds.) (1995). *Geriatric assessment technology: The state of the art.* New York: Springer.

Used with permission from Moorhead, S., et al. (2008). *Nursing outcomes classification (NOC)* (4th ed.), p. 530. St. Louis: Mosby.

---

2. Examples of nursing activities that would be appropriate for this patient include the following:
- Determine patient's readiness to engage in activity or exercise protocol.
- Collaborate with physical, occupational, and recreational therapists in developing and executing exercise program, as appropriate.
- Consult physical therapy to determine optimal position for patient during exercise and number of repetitions for each movement pattern.
- Explain rationale for type of exercise and protocol to patient/family.
- Sequence daily care activities to enhance effects of specific exercise therapy.
- Re-evaluate need for assistive devices at regular intervals in collaboration with PT, OT, or RT.
- Reorient patient to movement functions of the body.
- Assist patient to develop exercise protocol for strength, endurance, and flexibility.
- Incorporate ADLs into exercise protocol, if appropriate.
- Evaluate patient's progress toward enhancement/restoration of body movement and function.
  Note that other nursing activities may also be appropriate.

Out or in? Answers

1. Intervention
2. Outcome
3. Intervention
4. Intervention
5. Intervention
6. Outcome
7. Intervention
8. Intervention
9. Outcome
10. Outcome

Selected references

Ackley, B., & Ladwig, G. (2017). *Nursing diagnosis handbook: An evidenced-based guide to planning care* (11th Ed.). St. Louis, MO: Elsevier-Mosby.

Ballantyne, H. (2016). *Developing nursing care plans.* Retrieved on December 2016 from: http://journals.rcni.com/doi/pdfplus/10.7748/ns.30.26.51.s48

Bulechek, G., Butcher, H., Dochterman, J., & Wagner, C. (Eds.) (2013). Nursing interventions classification (NIC) (6th ed.). St. Louis, MO: Elsevier.

Hinkle, J., & Cheever, K. (2014). *Brunner & Suddarth's textbook of medical-surgical nursing* (13th Ed.). New York: Lippincott Williams & Wilkins.

Keenan, G., Yakel, E., Tschannen, D., & Mandeville, M. *Documentation and the nurse care planning process*. Retrieved on December 2016 from: https://www.ncbi.nlm.nih.gov/books/NBK2674/

Maas, M. L., & Specht, J. P. (2001). Impaired physical mobility. In M. Maas, K. Buckwalter, M. Hardy, T. Tripp-Reimer, M. Titler, & J. Specht (Eds.), *Nursing care of older adults: Diagnoses, outcomes & interventions* (pp. 337–365). St. Louis, MO: Mosby.

MJC Nursing Faculty (2012). *The nursing process assessment diagnosis planning/goal*. Retrieved on December 2016 from: https://www.mjc.edu/instruction/allied-health/adnprogram/nursingprocessoverview.pdf

Moorehead, S., Johson, M., Maas, M., & Swanson, E. (2013). *Nursing outcomes classification* (5th Ed.). St. Louis, MO: Elsevier-Mosby.

Nettina, S. (2014). *Lippincott's manual of nursing practice* (10th Ed.). New York: Lippincott Williams & Wilkins.

Podsiadlo, D., & Richardson, S. (1991). The timed "Up & Go": A test of basic functional mobility for frail elderly persons. *Journal of American Geriatrics Society, 39*(2), 142–148.

Rukenstein, L. Z., Wieland, D., & Bernakei, R. (Eds.). (1995). *Geriatric assessment technology: The state of the art*. New York: Springer.

Chapter 5

Implementation

Just the facts

In this chapter, you'll learn:

♦ responsibilities associated with implementation of a care plan

♦ strategies for gathering and organizing patient information

♦ methods for integrating safe and efficient patient care interventions

♦ the importance of communicating with the interprofessional health care team

♦ commonly used documentation methods

♦ patient safety goals promoted by the Joint Commission of Health Care Organizations (JCAHO)

Implementation overview

Once you've written a care plan—including the nursing diagnoses, patient outcomes, and interventions needed to achieve those outcomes—you're ready to put the care plan into action.

Less talk, more action. Implementation is the time to put your care plan into action.

Let's get hands-on

Implementation, the fourth step in the nursing process, is the step during which you'll have hands-on involvement with your patient. It encompasses:

• carrying out the planned interventions
• using your critical-thinking skills to solve problems and set priorities
• continually reassessing the patient's response to your interventions
• communicating effectively with other members of the health care team
• documenting all of the care you provide
• referral of patient to appropriate health care provider when needed.

All in a day's work

To implement a care plan, expect to perform some or all of the following types of interventions:

- conducting routine assessment and monitoring of the patient
- performing therapeutic interventions, such as administering medications or obtaining ordered specimens
- offering comfort measures
- providing nourishment
- helping with activities of daily living
- supporting respiratory and elimination functions
- providing skin care
- offering emotional support
- providing patient teaching and counseling
- communicating with interdisciplinary team members.

Somebody point me in the right direction!

It's normal to feel slightly overwhelmed and even frightened when you begin implementing your nursing care plan, especially if you're a nursing student or are just beginning your nursing career. However, this lack of confidence will dissipate with time and ongoing experience. Remember, the care plan is a road map to helping your patient achieve wellness. It will point you in the direction toward achieving that goal, but it's your responsibility to determine if you need additional information or need to collaborate with other health care team members before implementing an intervention.

Levels of responsibility

Your role in preparing and implementing a nursing care plan will vary with your level of nursing experience.

Student body

As a nursing student, your goal is to work from a care plan that you develop based on your assessment of the patient. In reality, you might not have access to your patient or his medical record until shortly before you become responsible for providing his care. In this situation, you need to review the care plan already in place as a blueprint for implementation. As you complete your own patient assessment, you become responsible for modifying the established care plan to reflect any changes and implementing your new interventions. The care plan you later write for your instructor may include diagnoses and interventions you actually had no time to initiate in the confines of your clinical time with the patient.

Don't be afraid to ask. If you need help, consult with other health care team members before you perform an intervention.

Nurse teamwork

As a practicing nurse, you'll initially follow a care plan developed by another nurse, and you may not know much about the patient before you actually meet him and begin providing care. Your game plan remains the same as when you were a student, though—modify the care plan as needed as you develop your own assessment data. As you're given new patients to admit to the unit, you'll have opportunities to develop complete care plans for them.

Regardless of your place in the nursing hierarchy, it's up to you to learn as much as you can about your patient and his current condition before implementing care. You're even responsible for making sure that a practitioner's orders are appropriate for a patient before you implement them.

Getting started

Start your implementation of the care plan by assessing the patient's current situation. Then gather the supplies you'll need to complete the planned interventions.

Assessing the situation

Even if this is your first encounter with this patient, a great deal of information about the patient is available to you from various sources. For example, you can gather plenty of useful information by:
- listening to the report of the departing nurse at the start of your shift
- reading the patient's medical record including information obtained during the initial history and physical examination
- talking with other staff, including your clinical instructor, the patient's primary nurse, and other members of the health care team
- talking with the patient and family members
- directly observing and assessing the patient
- reviewing laboratory and other test results.

Shifting gears

Begin your shift by listening to the previous shift nurse's report about the patient. (See *Electronic change-of-shift report at the bedside,* page 119.) On a work sheet, computer, or bedside workstation, document any pertinent information about the patient's vital signs, activities, intake and output, frequency of treatment, any medications given on an "as needed" basis and the patient's response, and special instructions, per the facility's guidelines.

Even after you graduate from student nurse to practicing nurse, your game plan should stay the same: Modify the care plan as needed as you develop your own assessment data.

Weighing the evidence

Electronic change-of-shift report at the bedside

The change-of-shift report is a time for nurses to communicate information about their patients to oncoming nurses for the next shift. They share such information as a patient's condition, status, signs and symptoms, medications, tests and test results, and response to medical interventions.

A study in 2012 examined nurse to nurse hand off of patient care at change of shift at the bedside of the patient. Findings indicated bedside nurse-to-nurse shift handoff had a positive impact on patients and nursing staff. Patients felt more informed of the plan of care for the day. Nurses' found there was more nurse-to-nurse accountability, medication reconciliation, and ability to communicate immediately with physicians regarding patient care. Staff nurses found bedside handoff a better way for them to prioritize the issues of patient care because they could visualize all their patients.

Source: Maxson, P. M., Derby, K. M., Wrobleski, D. M., & Foss, D. M. (2012). Bedside nurse to nurse handoff promotes patient safety. *Medsurg Nursing*, May/June 2012, 140–144; quiz 145.

If you work in a setting that has an electronic health record system, you may be able to print a patient-specific report of all orders and test results from the system. Some systems also contain the nursing care plans. (See *Sample electronic shift report*.)

Take note of this

After obtaining the report, you should review the patient's chart for any new orders that may have been prescribed. Note any changes in the patient's treatment or care regimen on both the care plan and your work sheet. Also review the medication and IV fluid administration record, and make notes (on your work sheet) of the times that medications, IV fluids, and other IV drugs are scheduled. Note the frequency of treatments, vital signs, dressing changes (and type), and blood glucose monitoring. This will help you to organize and integrate your planned independent nursing interventions with the collaborative interventions listed in the care plan.

Making contact

Next, assess the patient. After entering the patient's room, introduce yourself, wash your hands, and then check the patient's identification. Remember to use two patient identifiers, such as his name, birth date, or assigned identification number. Whenever possible, ask the patient to tell you his name instead of calling him by his name. (See *National Patient Safety Goals*, page 123.)

(*Text continues on page 122.*)

It's a good idea to highlight medication and IV administration times on your work sheet.

Sample electronic shift report

Many electronic health record systems are programmed to send practitioners' medical orders directly to the staff who will be implementing them. For example, new medication orders are sent to the pharmacy-specific section of the record system as well as to the nursing-specific section. Staff members in these departments can print out information they need to know from the records and use it to plan their work. Nurses usually obtain a printout (or electronic shift report) on each of their assigned patients at the start of their shifts. They might also regularly check the computer for new orders throughout their shift.

Although electronic shift reports are valuable, they shouldn't be used in place of verbal shift reports because the data they provide about a patient's current status are limited. For example, electronic reports don't tell you how your patient is doing, what issues are most important for follow-up, or what the previous assessment revealed. The electronic shift report printout is a good place to make notes about information obtained during the verbal shift report.

Here's a sample electronic nursing shift report.

Sample electronic shift report (*continued*)

```
Medical ICU-4321              Patient Care Hospital
3/14/12     07:00             PAGE 002
=================================================================

WILLIAMS, HENRY               66  MWMC
MR#: 5555555      DOB 10/26/40  MICU 302
FIN#: 1010101010              Admitted: 3/12/12
DR: Daniel Smith             Service: Internal Medicine
=================================================================

Summary: 3/14 07:00 to 15:00

NURSE COMMUNICATIONS:
3/12/12      IV site Right arm #20 inserted, restart on
             3/15/12

ALL CURRENT MEDICAL ORDERS
Doctor to Nurse Orders:
3/12/12      Blood cultures x 2 if temperature > 101  F,
             Nurse please enter as a secondary order,
             when necessary.
3/12/12      Cardiology: ECG 12 lead Stat, prn chest
             pain, Nurse please enter as a secondary
             order, when necessary.
3/12/12      Sequential Teds: Patient to wear continuous-
             ly while in bed.
3/12/12      Foley catheter to urometer, measure output
             q 1 hour, notify MD if UO < 30 ml/hour or >
             300 ml/hour x 2 hours.
3/12/12      Notify MD for SBP > 180 mm Hg or < 110 mm
             Hg
3/12/12      Notify MD for change in mental status
3/12/12      Accucheck q 6 hours

Vital Sign Orders:
3/12/12      VS: q 1 hour with neurological checks

Diet:
3/12/12      Diet: NPO

I&O Orders:
3/12/12      Per ICU routine

Activity:
3/12/12      Activity: Bedrest with HOB elevated 30
             degrees
IVS:
3/12/12      IV line Dextrose 5% & Sodium Chloride 0.45%
             1000 ml, Rate: 80 ml/hour, x 2 bags

Scheduled Medications:
3/12/12      Decadron Dexamethasone Inj 4 mg, IV, q 6
             hours
                  09       15
```

The current medical orders are broken down into categories. In shift report, note the status of each order and the latest assessment results. Leave space for your assessments.

(*continued*)

Sample electronic shift report (*continued*)

```
Medical ICU-4321              Patient Care Hospital
3/14/12      07:00            PAGE 003
================================================================

WILLIAMS, HENRY                  66  MWMC
MR#: 5555555      DOB 10/26/40   MICU 302
FIN#: 1010101010                 Admitted: 3/12/12
DR: Daniel Smith                 Service: Internal Medicine
================================================================

Summary: 3/14 07:00 to 15:00

3/12/12          Lopressor Metoprolol Inj 5 mg, IV, q 6
                 hours
                     09        15
3/12/12          Heparin inj 5,000 units, SC, q 12 hours
                     09

Miscellaneous Medications:
3/13/12          Lasix Furosemide Inj 40 mg, IV, Now

PRN Medications:
3/12/12          Tylenol Acetaminophen Supp 650 mg, #1, PR,
                 q 4 hour prn pain or temperature > 101 F

Laboratory:
3/14/12          Basic metabolic panel tomorrow, collect at
                 05:00
3/14/12          CBC/Diff/Plts tomorrow, collect at 05:00
3/14/12          Cardiac troponin, tomorrow, collect at 05:00

Radiology:
3/12/12          Computed tomography: CT scan of the head
                 without contrast STAT

Ancillary:
3/12/12          Respiratory care: Oxygen via nasal cannula
                 at 2L/minute.
3/12/12          Physical therapy: Patient evaluation and
                 treatment
                          Last page
```

> For diagnostic and laboratory tests, verify that the reports are in the chart and check the results.

Perform your initial assessment and make notes of your findings; these notes will provide the basis for your initial nurse's note in the patient's medical record. You can also use this opportunity to talk briefly with the patient (and any family members who may be present if the patient gives permission) and gather additional information about the patient's:

- perception of his current illness and his overall health and well-being
- ability to perform the interventions to meet the outcomes specified in the care plan
- available resources and support system.

Weighing the evidence

National Patient Safety Goals

Since July 2002, The Joint Commission has annually published National Patient Safety Goals that they require an organization to meet before it can be accredited. These standards, or goals, are developed based on safety statistics, research, and input from numerous health care professionals and consumers.

A few of the important safety goals you might need to implement in your clinical settings are:
- Use at least two patient identifiers when providing care, treatment, and services.
- Eliminate transfusion errors related to patient misidentification.
- Report critical results of tests and diagnostic procedures on a timely basis.
- Label all medications, medication containers, and other solutions on and off the sterile field in perioperative and other procedural settings.
- Reduce the likelihood of patient harm associated with the use of anticoagulant therapy.
- Maintain and communicate accurate patient medication information.
- Improve the safety of clinical alarm systems.
- Comply with either the current Centers for Disease Control and Prevention (CDC) hand hygiene guidelines or the current World Health Organization (WHO) hand hygiene guidelines.
- Implement evidence-based practices to prevent central line–associated blood-stream infections.
- Implement evidence-based practices for preventing surgical site infections.
- Implement evidence-based practices to prevent indwelling catheter-associated urinary tract infections (CAUTI).
- Identify patients at risk for suicide.
- Use the universal protocol for preventing wrong site, wrong procedure, and wrong person surgery.

Source: For a complete list of patient safety goals see: The Joint Commission. National Patient Safety Goals. Available at www.jointcommission.org/PatientSafety/NationalPatientSafetyGoals/

Student report

If you're a student, provide a brief verbal report of your findings to the patient's assigned nurse and your clinical instructor, alerting them immediately to any abnormal findings. Ask them to clarify anything you're unsure about or ask your clinical instructor to check on the patient to verify your findings. (See *Nurses as resources*.)

Nurses as resources

Experienced nurses can be invaluable resources. They've amassed a wealth of information through practical experience in providing bedside care. They can teach you organizational skills and strategies for thinking through situations that you may encounter in the clinical setting. Tapping into their knowledge can help you to fine-tune your assessment and care techniques in your quest to become a registered nurse.

Gathering supplies

After you've performed your initial assessment, you'll gather and assemble the appropriate equipment and supplies for other interventions you'll need to perform. Once you've properly prepared yourself and the necessary supplies, it's time to implement patient care.

Providing care

Now, you're ready to begin tackling specific interventions. Being prepared and developing a system that integrates various activities can save you time and benefit your patient by reducing interruptions to his rest.

Make sure that you have the right drug, dose, patient, time, and route.

Basic implementation steps

Although the specific care activities that you'll perform will depend on the patient's condition, some general practices apply to all patients. The timing of meals, therapies, tests, and procedures the patient is scheduled to receive will determine which of the other interventions specified in the care plan you'll initiate next.

Meet Mr. Med

When your patient is due to receive a medication, locate and prepare the medications under the supervision of your nursing instructor or the patient's primary nurse. (See *Safe drug administration guidelines*, page 125.) Follow a tried-and-true set of safeguards known as the "Rights of Medication Administration" to help you avoid the most

Safe drug administration guidelines

When administering a drug, be sure to adhere to best practices to avoid potential problems and manage those that do occur. You can help prevent drug errors by following these guidelines as well as facility policy.

Drug orders

- Don't rely on the pharmacy computer system to detect all unsafe orders. Before you give a drug, understand the correct dosage, indications, and adverse effects.
- Be aware of the drugs your patient takes regularly, and question any deviation from his regular routine. As with any drug, take your time and read the label carefully.
- Before you give drugs that are ordered in units, such as insulin and heparin, always check the prescriber's written order against the provided dose. Never abbreviate the word "units."
- To prevent an acetaminophen overdose from combined analgesics, note the amount of acetaminophen in each drug. Beware of substitutions by the pharmacy because the amount of acetaminophen may vary.

Drug preparation and administration

- Always check the expiration date before administering a drug.
- If a familiar drug has an unfamiliar appearance, find out why. If the pharmacist cites a manufacturing change, ask him to double-check whether he has received verification from the manufacturer. Document the appearance discrepancy, your actions, and the pharmacist's response in the patient record.
- Use two patient identifiers, such as the patient's name and assigned identification number, to identify the patient before administering any drug or treatment. Teach the patient to offer his identification bracelet for inspection when anyone arrives with drugs and to insist on having it replaced if it's removed.
- Ask the patient to verify his allergy history before administering an antibiotic.
- Ask the patient about his use of alternative therapies, including herbs, and record your findings in his medical record. Monitor the patient carefully and report unusual events. Ask the patient to keep a diary of all therapies he uses and to take the diary for review each time he visits a health care professional.

- If your facility uses a bar code administration system, follow the manufacturer's and your facility's policies for use. Normal: Never bypass safety protocols.

Avoiding common problems
Calculation errors

- Writing the milligrams per kilogram (mg/kg) or milligrams per meter squared (mg/m^2) dose and the calculated dose provides a safeguard against calculation errors. Whenever a prescriber provides the calculation, double-check it and document that the dose was verified.
- Don't assume that liquid drugs are less likely to cause harm than other forms. Pediatric and geriatric patients commonly receive liquid drugs and may be especially sensitive to the effects of an inaccurate dose. If a unit-dose form isn't available, calculate carefully and double-check your math and the drug label.
- Have another nurse verify your calculations, especially insulin and heparin dosages and calculations.
- Read the label on every drug you prepare and never administer any drug that is ambiguously labeled or difficult to read.

Air bubbles in pump tubing

- To clear bubbles from IV tubing, never increase the pump's flow rate to flush the line. Instead, remove the tubing from the pump, disconnect it from the patient, and use the flow control clamp to establish gravity flow.
- When the bubbles have been removed, return the tubing to the pump, restart the infusion, and recheck the flow rate.

Incorrect administration route

- When a patient has multiple IV lines, label the distal end of each line.
- Never use a parenteral syringe to prepare oral liquid drugs (this increases the chance for error because the syringe tip fits easily into IV ports). To safely give an oral drug through a feeding tube, use a dose prepared by the pharmacy and a syringe with the appropriate tip.

basic and common medication errors. Each time you administer a medication, confirm that you have the:

- right patient
- right medication
- right dosage
- right time
- right route
- right documentation
- right reason
- right response.

Room service

At meal times, raise the head of the bed so that the patient can sit upright. Adjust his tray, and assess his need for fresh water. Ask about any special requests, such as the desire for juice or other food items. Place the call light within the patient's reach, and instruct him to call you with any additional needs or concerns.

Before you leave

Each time you prepare to exit the patient's room review your care plan and work sheet. Identify the interventions you've completed, and make note of any changes to the care plan that need to be made. Also document any changes in the patient's status, his response to treatment and care, or his refusal of care, all treatments, and regimens (all of which require nursing documentation in the patient's medical record).

Status report

Report any abnormal findings, patient or family concerns, changes in the patient's condition, or uncertainty or concern about findings to your clinical instructor and the patient's primary care nurse. Also report and document completion of ordered treatments and regimens.

Integrating activities

Although you could approach each intervention separately when providing care, systematically checking off each intervention in the care plan, this approach isn't the most practical use of your time and energy. A more effective approach is to try completing as many interventions as possible during each visit to the patient's room. Coordinating and integrating your nursing care between or with activities of daily living, medication administration, vital signs assessments,

Memory jogger

Before you administer a drug, remember your nursing responsibilities for this intervention. To remember the sequence of the actions you must take, think "Until Clear, Ask Many Times":

UCAMT

Understand the drug and how it works.

Clarify the drug order as needed.

Administer the drug.

Monitor the patient for response to the drug and for adverse effects.

Teach the patient about the drug as needed.

treatments, and other collaborative and interdependent care has several benefits:

- It saves time.
- It lessens the interruptions of patient rest.
- It allows you to provide efficient and timely care.

When taking an integrated approach, remember to review your care plan and documentation carefully because you'll be attempting to complete several interventions during a single visit.

Implementation example

Because the care that you provide is specific to each patient, a sample scenario might help you to better understand ways in which you can successfully integrate routine activities to implement efficient patient care. Suppose you're working the morning shift (7 AM to 3 PM) in a hospital and you're assigned a patient with a neuromuscular impairment. After report, you review the care plan, which included the nursing diagnoses:

- *Bathing self-care deficit related to neuromuscular impairment and generalized debility as evidenced by inability to wash body and obtain bath supplies*
- *Risk for impaired skin integrity related to decreased mobility and poor nutritional intake.*

Your nursing care plan for this patient might look like the one shown in *Understanding implementation: Sample care plan.*

Based on the care plan, interventions for this patient may include:

- taking vital signs
- assisting with morning hygiene (such as bathing, oral care, toileting, and grooming)
- assessing skin, diet, fluid intake, musculoskeletal strength, and mobility
- positioning the patient
- providing nutritious meals.

You'll also need to incorporate other assessments, such as assessment of cardiopulmonary status, bowel elimination, and pain, into your care to gain a full picture of the patient's status.

Making the most of your time

Remember, to provide the most efficient care possible, you may need to integrate several interventions. Here are some ways in which you can integrate the nursing tasks that you need to perform:

- If the patient's ability allows, ask him to wash his face while you're setting up supplies for his bed bath. Observe the patient's reaction and the action taken in response to this request. Assess the patient's interest in self-care, ability to understand and follow instructions, functional use and range of motion (ROM) of upper extremities, and any signs of discomfort.

- While the patient washes himself, ask about pain or discomfort with movement, level of fatigue, usual activity level before this hospitalization, the availability of people to assist him at home, and any preferences for skin care.
- While helping the patient shave, assess endurance and fine motor skills and ROM of the hands and arms.
- When applying lotion to the patient's hands, assess bilateral grip strength, radial pulses, capillary refill, and gross sensory disturbances.
- While washing the patient's lower extremities, assess strength and ROM of legs and feet, endurance, skin integrity, distal pulses, capillary refill, toenails, and gross sensory disturbances.
- While helping the patient wash his perineal area, discuss bowel and bladder status or problems and observe skin integrity of the abdomen and groin.
- While assisting with oral hygiene, assess the teeth, gums, tongue, and oral mucosa and encourage the patient to drink sufficient amounts of water. Teach the importance of adequate fluid intake to maintain healthy skin and bowel and bladder function.

Mealtimes are another good opportunity to assess your patient's status and his needs.

Working with the interprofessional team

Nurses aren't the only health care professionals involved in patient care. As you implement care, you'll need to collaborate with an interprofessional team to meet the diverse needs of your patients.

Share and share alike

The focus of an interprofessional team is on the patient and patient outcomes. Each team member shares responsibility for achieving these outcomes. To provide more effective and comprehensive care, you need to understand each team member's role. (See *Meet the interdisciplinary team*, page 131.)

Remember, patient care is a team sport.

Passing notes is permitted

When you're reviewing the patient's chart, be sure to read documentation written by other members of the health care team. Those notes will provide you with important information about your patient's treatment and progress toward outcomes.

If you have questions about the patient's condition or treatment, contact the appropriate team members for more information. For example, a pharmacist can tell you how to space medications to eliminate drug or food interactions, whereas a physical therapist can provide you with written instructions on the patient's prescribed exercises.

(*Text continues on page 131.*)

Understanding implementation: Sample care plan

This sample care plan was developed for a patient who has problems with bathing and hygiene and who's at risk for skin breakdown because of his chronic illness and current hospitalization.

Date	Nursing diagnosis	Patient outcomes	Interventions	Outcome evaluation (initials and date)
5/8/17	Bathing self-care deficit related to neuromuscular impairment and generalized debility as evidenced by inability to wash body and obtain bath supplies	• The patient will wash his face, arms, frontal trunk, and perineal area on morning shift by discharge. • The family will demonstrate safe and effective assistance with patient's bath and hygiene on morning shift by discharge.	• Assess the patient's functional level every shift, and document findings. • Assist with or perform bathing daily while promoting patient independence in bathing the parts of his body within his reach and his maximal functional ability. • Change linens daily and as needed. • Assess the family's knowledge of proper bath and linen change procedures, safety measures, and rationale for personal hygiene in order to meet the patient's bathing and hygiene needs on discharge. • Instruct the family as needed on safe techniques for providing bathing and hygiene needs. • Observe family members demonstrate safe and effective assistance with the patient's personal care. • Assess the family's need for home care assistance to provide the patient's bathing and hygiene needs for safety or respite issues.	

REVIEW DATES

Date	Signature	Initials
5/8/17	Jackie Miller, RN	JM

Understanding implementation: Sample care plan (*continued*)

Date	Nursing diagnosis	Patient outcomes	Interventions	Outcome evaluation (initials and date)
5/8/17	Risk for impaired skin integrity related to decreased mobility and poor nutritional intake	• The patient will remain free from skin break-down during the hospital stay. • The patient will consume 80% of all meals during hospital stay. • The family will dem-onstrate proper use and under-standing of home mea-sures to prevent skin breakdown by discharge.	• Assess skin integrity every shift and as needed. • Assess dietary and fluid pref-erences on admission. • Assess dietary intake and fluid intake and output every shift. • Assess the family's knowledge of principles and practices of skin care and their need for specialized equipment to pro-mote good care at home. • Keep skin and linens clean and dry, and keep linens wrin-kle-free. • Turn and reposition the patient every 2 hours and as needed. • Apply lotion to dry skin areas after bathing, at bedtime, and as desired by the patient. • Provide foods and fluids of choice that are nutritionally appropriate for the patient's diet and medical regimen. • Promote patient intake of at least 1 L of noncaffeinated liq-uids per day. • Teach the family as needed about skin care and observa-tion techniques, position change requirements, and nutritional and fluid needs to prevent skin breakdown. • Observe the family demonstrate and verbalize understanding of all instructions given.	

REVIEW DATES		
Date	Signature	Initials
5/8/17	Jackie Miller, RN	JM

Meet the interdisciplinary team

Members of the interdisciplinary health care team—and their roles—include:
- physician, physician's assistant, nurse practitioner, and consultant specialty physicians—who assess, monitor, and provide treatment guidelines for the patient's medical conditions
- primary nurse, advanced practice or clinical nurse specialist, and nurse-manager—who assess, monitor, teach, and intervene to help the patient meet his expected outcomes by discharge
- registered dietitian—who assesses and monitors nutritional needs
- social worker—who provides support and counseling to patients and their families and helps with financial difficulties
- occupational therapist—who assists the patient in performing activities of daily living, participating in recreation, and working to the highest functional level
- physical therapist—who assists the patient to improve or restore physical functioning and prevent deconditioning
- respiratory therapist—who monitors and provides airway management and oxygenation
- pastoral care specialist—who provides religious and spiritual support to patients and their families
- pharmacist—who reviews, prepares, and dispenses the patient's medications; provides information and guidance in the preparation and administration of medications; and provides patient education (in an outpatient setting)
- case manager—who coordinates access to ongoing services after discharge, such as transfer to another facility, arrangement for medical equipment in the home, or referral for home health services.

Hospice or palliative care

In a hospice or palliative care setting, the interdisciplinary team would also include:
- volunteer—who provides emotional and diversional support and respite to the patient and family
- bereavement counselor—who supports and counsels the family for 1 year after the death of the patient.

Important reminder

And don't forget the most important members of the team: the patient and his family.
   No interventions can occur and no goals can be met unless the patient permits the care and is committed to the outcome.

Play well with others

You'll also need to coordinate care with other team members. For example, medicating your postoperative patient before respiratory exercises helps the patient cough and deep breathe more effectively with the respiratory therapist. When working with other team members, remember to use good communication skills. Above all, treat all team members with respect, and they'll respect you in turn!

Documenting interventions

Documentation is an important component of implementation. As previously mentioned, you should take notes after each intervention you perform, including the nature of the intervention, the time you performed it, and the patient's response as well as interventions you performed based on the patient's response and the reasons you performed them. Each intervention should also be documented in the patient's medical record. You should record interventions whenever you:

- perform routine care
- perform emergency care
- observe changes in the patient's condition
- administer medications
- perform procedures or interventions.

Tailor-fit to house style

Where do you document your interventions? That depends on your facility's policy. You can document them on graphic records, on a patient care flow sheet that integrates all nurses' notes for a 1-day period, on integrated or separate nurses' progress notes, and on other specialized documentation forms (such as the medication administration record). Your facility's policies also dictate the style and format of the documentation.

Focused documentation

Your documentation should be patient centered and outcome oriented. Stating the patient's response to your nursing interventions help to make your documentation patient centered. Linking your interventions and responses to the nursing diagnoses and goal statements makes it outcome oriented as well.

Documentation formats

Various types of nursing documentation formats are used in the clinical setting. They may be done by hand or in a computerized charting system. Two of the most commonly used formats for documenting interventions are discussed here.

PIE system

The problem-intervention-evaluation (PIE) system organizes information according to patient problems and was devised to simplify the documentation process. This system requires you to keep a daily patient assessment flow sheet and to write structured progress notes.

Piecing PIE together

Each piece of PIE has it's own purpose:
- The problem category is used to identify the nursing diagnosis requiring the interventions.
- The intervention category describes the actions you took and any assessment data related to the interventions.
- The evaluation section describes the results of your interventions and any additional information regarding attaining your outcomes. (See *Using PIE documentation.*)

SOAP format

SOAP is an acronym for subjective data, objective data, assessment, and planning. The SOAP system, which is used in problem-oriented medical record charting, allows all health care team members to record their findings using narrative progress notes. This system allows readers to readily distinguish between the subjective and objective data so the correct plan of care can be chosen, and you can show that your interventions addressed the patient's documented needs. It also specifies the follow-up care that's planned.

The dirt on SOAP

To use the SOAP format, document the following information for each problem:
- Subjective data: Information the patient or family members tell you, such as the chief complaint
- Objective data: Factual, measurable data you gather during assessment, such as vital signs and laboratory test results
- Assessment data: Conclusions based on the collected subjective and objective data and formulated as patient problems and nursing diagnoses; these conclusions are dynamic, changing as more or different data become known
- Plan: Your strategy for relieving the patient's problem, including both short- and long-term measures. (See *Using SOAP notes.*)

Using PIE documentation

For the nursing diagnosis *Bathing self-care deficit,* you would document your care using the PIE format in this way:

P—Bathing self-care deficit

I—Assisted pt. with bath; he was able to wash his own hands and upper chest slowly without discomfort. Pt. unable to lift arms above chest; muscle strength grade 3/6 upper and lower extremities.

Remains on practitioner-ordered bed rest. Changed linens and repositioned pt. onto left side after applying oil-based lotion to skin.

E—Continues to require major assistance with personal care. Plan to assess the family's ability to meet the pt.'s bathing and hygiene needs when they visit in the afternoon.

For the nursing diagnosis *Risk for impaired skin integrity,* you would document your care using the PIE format in this way:

P—Risk for impaired skin integrity

I—Pt. assessment revealed warm, dry skin that's papery on the lower legs with some flaking. Sacral area is reddened from lying supine, but color clears when the patient is repositioned onto left side. No other areas of redness or any other defects present. Radial, dorsalis pedis, and posterior tibial pulses +2 and equal bilaterally; all nail beds show brisk capillary refill. Applied lotion after bath. Pt. ate 50% of breakfast; states "I don't get too hungry anymore." I like a hot breakfast but "I don't care for bacon or sausage, just eggs or oatmeal". Instructed pt. that dietitian can visit and help him choose meals he likes as well as find ways to keep up his protein and calories so his skin remains healthy. Pt. agreeable but requests visit in the afternoons, when his wife is here. Also taught pt. importance of drinking 4 to 6 cups of noncaffeinated fluids per day for skin, bowel, and bladder health and applying lotion to dry extremities, particularly the lower legs, at least twice daily. E—Pt. verbalized understanding of all instructions but prefers to have wife hear information as well; pt. states "she keeps track of everything now." Pt. offers to ask her to rub lotion on his legs and arms during her afternoon visits. Referral made to dietitian.

Using SOAP notes

For the patient problem *Bathing self-care deficit,* you would document your care using the SOAP format in this way:

> S—"I can't get to my bath supplies because my strength is gone.
> I can't even move myself."
> O—Pt. unable to lift arms above chest. Washed own hands and upper chest slowly. Muscle strength grade 3/6 upper and lower extremities. Pt. remains on practitioner-ordered bed rest.
> A—Bathing self-care deficit
> P—Continue to provide for pt.'s bathing and hygiene needs. Assess and instruct family regarding alternate methods for meeting bathing and hygiene needs.

For the patient problem *Risk for impaired skin integrity,* you would document your care using the SOAP format in this way:

> S—"I'm feeling some pressure and pain in my lower back."
> O—Papery dry skin on the lower legs with some flaking; sacral area reddened from lying supine.
> A—Risk for impaired skin integrity
> P—Continue to change position frequently. Apply lotion to dry areas.

SBAR documentation format

In 2012, to enhance patient safety, the Joint Commission has recommended the SBAR (Situation, Background, Assessment, Recommendation) communication format. SBAR can be applied to many forms of communication between healthcare providers and provides a standard framework for transfer of information. SBAR is particularly effective:

- when nurses need to call other health care providers, such as physicians, on the telephone
- during change of shift, when there is handoff of patient responsibilities to another nurse or other health care provider
- when transferring patients to other organizations or levels of care.

   S = Situation (a concise statement of the problem; clearly and briefly define the situation)

   B = Background (pertinent and relevant history information related to the patient and situation)

A = Assessment (analysis and considerations of options—what you found/think)

R = Recommendation (action requested/recommended—what you want)

The following is an example of SBAR used between a home health care nurse and physician.

Situation: This is Mary Remington, a home health care nurse taking care of "Mr. Robert Smith who is being treated for deep venous thrombosis. The patient has two prescriptions for Coumadin and he is unclear as to which one he is supposed to take."

Background: The patient is a 78-year-old male with DVT who was discharged from the hospital on June 5 and sent home with a prescription for Coumadin 2 mg po once a day. On a follow-up with an office visit with Dr. White on June 7, he was prescribed Coumadin 5 mg po once a day.

Assessment: The patient needs clarity about the proper dosage of Coumadin to take daily.

Recommendation: Please clarify which is the correct dose of Coumadin for Mr. Jones to take and which physician is managing his anticoagulant therapy.

On the case

Case study background

For your first clinical rotation on a medical-surgical unit, you're assigned to care for two patients. Your first patient is Shirley Trotter, a 75-year-old who was admitted yesterday with pneumonia and severe shortness of breath. Your second patient is Carl Conrad, a 46-year-old admitted 3 days ago for an abdominal cholecystectomy.

Critical thinking exercise

To help prepare for your clinical experience, place these steps in proper sequence by numbering them from 1 to 10:

A. Assess Shirley Trotter.

B. Document your care and the patients' responses to your interventions.

C. Receive the shift report from your patients' previous nurse.

D. Greet your patients, introduce yourself to them, and verify their identities per protocol.

E. Check in with your instructor and prepare the patients' morning medications, gathering any other supplies needed.

F. Receive your patient assignment, research the medical diagnoses and existing care plans, and establish preliminary priorities of care.
G. Assess Carl Conrad.
H. Review medication and IV fluid administration records.
I. Complete as many interventions as possible during each visit to each patient's room.
J. Administer your patients' morning medications.

Answer key

Critical thinking exercise

1. F, 2. C, 3. H, 4. D, 5. A, 6. G, 7. E, 8. J, 9. I, 10. B

Selected references

2017 National Patient Safety Goals. Available at: https://www.jointcommission.org/standards_information/npsgs.aspx

American Nurses Association. (2015). *Nursing: Scope and standards of practice* (3rd ed.). Silver Spring, MD: American Nurses Association.

Buchholz, S. (2016). *Med-math*. Philadelphia, PA: Wolters Kluwer.

Maxson, P. M., Derby, K. M., Wrobleski, D. M., & Foss, D. M. (2012). Bedside nurse-to-nurse handoff promotes patient safety. *Medsurg Nursing, 21*(3), 140–145.

Taylor, C., & Lillis, P. (2014). *Fundamentals of nursing: The art and science of person-centered nursing care* (8th ed.). Philadelphia, PA: Lippincott Williams & Wilkins.

Wilkinson, J. M., Treas, L. S., Barnett, K. L., & Smith, M. H. (2016). *Fundamentals of nursing volume 1: Theory, concepts, and applications* (3rd ed.). Philadelphia, PA: F.A. Davis.

Chapter 6

Evaluation

Just the facts

In this chapter, you'll learn:

◆ the importance of continually reassessing the patient's condition during all phases of care

◆ criteria for evaluating care

◆ the process for evaluating whether a care plan must be revised and the way in which revisions should be implemented.

A look at evaluation

Although designated as the fifth phase of the nursing process, evaluation is really an ongoing practice that occurs with every patient encounter. It encompasses:

- reassessing the patient
- comparing your findings with the outcome criteria established in the care plan
- determining the extent of the patient's progress, or outcome achievement (whether an outcome goal was met, partially met, or not met)
- writing evaluation statements
- revising the care plan, including nursing diagnoses, outcomes, and interventions, as needed
- documenting your evaluation.

The value of evaluation

Each evaluation you make depends primarily on your ability to form an opinion or judgment about the data you collect. As a nurse, you'll use your evaluation findings to:

- determine if the original assessment findings still apply to the patient's condition
- uncover complications
- assess and analyze trends or patterns in the patient's response to all aspects of his or her care, including medications, changes in diet or activity, procedures, unusual incidents or problems, and teaching

Don't be nervous about being evaluated. Evaluation is an ongoing and critical part of patient care.

- determine how closely your care conforms to established standards
- assess the results of care provided by other health care team members
- identify opportunities to improve the quality of care.

Reassessing a patient

Reassessment is a necessary part of evaluation. After all, how else can you determine whether your patient's condition is improving, your interventions are working, or your patient is making sufficient progress toward achieving outcome goals?

The patient and the process

It's important to note that reassessment includes not only periodically rechecking your patient's status throughout his care but also reexamining all phases of the nursing process in relation to the patient. This involves reviewing all the nursing diagnoses, patient outcomes, and specific interventions written into the care plan. (See *Evaluation throughout the nursing process.*)

Reassessment is a necessary part of evaluation.

Evaluation throughout the nursing process

Assessment, or more correctly *reassessment,* takes place at all phases of the nursing process. Examples of the types of questions you can ask as you move through the stages of the nursing process are shown below. Remember that any change in the patient's condition that's outside of the expected findings requires you to notify the practitioner.

Nursing process step		Questions
Assessment		Have the patient's vital signs changed? What's the patient's current pain scale rating?
Nursing diagnosis		Is this diagnosis still relevant? Do the current signs and symptoms point to any new diagnoses?
Planning		Are the outcomes still realistic in the time allotted? Do the interventions still match the patient's expected outcomes?
Implementation		Did I observe a response when I implemented the interventions? Was the patient comfortable with the interventions?
Evaluation		How do the reassessment findings compare with the original findings? Can I document the patient's expected outcome as met?

Comparing patient data

In order to evaluate care, you must first compare your patient's prior assessment data with your follow-up assessment data to see whether the patient's condition has changed. This comparison allows you to make inferences about the patient's condition and to alter the care plan accordingly.

Data déjà vu

When comparing data, remember to review all the patient's findings, including:
- the patient's baseline level of functioning at the time of admission
- the patient's most recent assessment findings
- any other pertinent data collected within the past 24 hours.

Your comparison should include a careful review of the patient's functional level, vital signs, and general overall status.

Begging the question

Next, you should compare the patient's current condition with condition prior to the initiation of care to determine the patient's response to your interventions (independent and collaborative). Ask yourself these two key questions:

How is my patient responding to care?

What's my patient's current condition (stable, improving, or worsening)?

Your answers to these questions will help guide your decisions about follow-up care. (For an example of how to evaluate patient data, see *Is my patient improving?* page 141.)

Report, record, react

The follow-up care you'll perform will be determined by the results of your reassessment evaluation. If the patient's condition is stable or improved, your next step is documentation of your findings. If, however, you believe that the patient's condition is remaining static or deteriorating, be prepared to suggest the next appropriate actions and give your rationales for them. Then proceed with further interventions as appropriate. Keep in mind that you'll need to document your findings and the care plan revisions. As a student nurse, you'll also need to report your assessment data to the primary nurse and your instructor.

Is my patient improving?

You've been working with an elderly, bedbound, terminally ill patient. One of the major nursing considerations for this patient is his comfort level, which includes keeping him free from painful skin breakdown.

Initial assessment

The patient's initial assessment showed:
- very dry, flaking skin on the lower legs and feet
- buildup of dead skin on the soles
- deep-red heels that are continuously tender
- present and equal dorsalis pedis and posterior tibial pulses bilaterally
- absence of edema
- sluggish capillary refill.

A nursing diagnosis of *Impaired skin integrity related to immobility, decreased nutrition, and skin effects of aging* was identified on the patient's care plan, which also included the following expected outcomes:
- The skin on the patient's lower extremities will be pink, dry, and intact by discharge.
- The patient's skin will be free from additional areas of impaired skin integrity throughout hospitalization.

Your assessment

Your assessment on day 3 of admission reveals:
- soft skin on the lower legs and feet
- slight flaking of the skin on the ankles and feet
- decrease of 50% in residual dead skin buildup
- deep-red heels that are tender to touch
- unchanged pulses, edema, and capillary refill.

Comparing assessments

When you compare the new data you collected with the initial patient data, you determine that the patient's condition is improving and your plan is to continue to implement the nursing interventions identified on the care plan and to continue to monitor the patient. If your assessment had revealed that the patient's condition was unstable or worsening, in addition to continuing with established interventions you may add new interventions, such as consulting the practitioner and wound care specialist for additional treatments or requesting an order for a specialty bed.

Keeping track of interventions

One suggestion for keeping track of the interventions you perform is to check off the interventions after you perform them, and then write down data that suggest the patient is making progress toward achieving the goal. Also remember to evaluate and document in your notes how the patient tolerates the interventions you perform and any unexpected effects related to the intervention.

Evaluating interventions and goals

At some point, you'll need to conduct a systematic review of all your interventions to gauge your patient's progress toward achieving the expected outcomes. When you do this, you'll ask yourself many additional questions, such as:

- Do the reassessment findings show that the interventions are working?
- Are some interventions no longer necessary?
- Have any or all of the patient's short-term goals been met? Have long-term goals been met?

Complete or communicate

As a student, you might not be able to perform all of the interventions included in a patient's care plan. However, you're responsible for communicating to your instructor and the patient's primary care nurse which interventions you did and did not complete. (See *Keeping track of interventions.*) This communication ensures that the patient's primary care nurse knows what interventions still need to be completed so that the patient receives all of the planned nursing interventions.

Achieving expected outcomes

On evaluation, you may determine, based on the patient's response to treatment and care, that the patient has met short-term goals. For example, you may have successfully employed all of the interventions needed to return your patient's assessment findings to within normal limits. Hence, your evaluation would lead you to assume that the expected outcome has been met.

To help clarify this concept, consider a practical real-life example, such as preparing a low-calorie dinner. (See *Dinner with friends*, page 143.)

Dinner with friends

Here's a practical example of how to evaluate whether expected outcomes have been met: Imagine that you are preparing dinner for some friends. Your friends are all watching their calories and request a low-calorie meal. You have all your ingredients except for low-calorie salad dressing. Your nursing diagnosis is (*not a NANDA-I diagnosis*) *Salad dressing deficit.* Your short-term goal is to go to the grocery store to purchase low-calorie salad dressing. You drive to the nearby supermarket and see a wide selection of different dressings. You decide to purchase low-calorie Ranch dressing.

So, from a nursing perspective, how would you evaluate what you've just done? In this example, the best approach is to compare the diagnosis with the goal to determine what you've accomplished.

When expected outcomes aren't met

Achieving expected outcomes indicates progress in your patient's care. However, suppose that you perform all of the interventions in the care plan and your patient's condition doesn't improve or, worse yet, has deteriorated. These findings indicate that the expected outcomes haven't been achieved. So, what do you do? At this point, you must reassess the situation.

A case of intolerable interventions?

You're caring for a 78-year-old patient with a nursing diagnosis of *Toileting self-care deficit related to weakness as evidenced by muscle strength 4/6 in lower extremities, a prior order for bed rest, and loss of muscle mass due to aging.* This patient's expected outcome is that he will ambulate

Positive outcomes indicate progress!

to the bathroom with assistance the 3rd day after admission. You begin performing the following interventions, as mentioned in the care plan:

- Assess the patient's functional level and strength before getting him out of bed.
- Dangle the patient's feet at the side of the bed before assisting him to a standing position.
- Assist the patient out of bed to the bathroom when needed.
- Instruct the patient to call for assistance with toileting before an urgent need, and explain planned interventions to achieve the expected outcome.

As soon as you begin assisting the patient to sit on the side of the bed to dangle his legs, you hear him state that he feels dizzy. You immediately help him to lie back down in bed and take these vital signs: blood pressure 80/58 mm Hg, pulse 110 beats/minute, and oxygen saturation per pulse oximetry 97% on room air. You check these measurements and find that the patient's morning vital signs were blood pressure 110/64 mm Hg, pulse 88 beats/minute, and oxygen saturation per pulse oximetry 97% on room air. These vital sign changes and the patient's complaint of dizziness lead you to conclude that the patient's condition has changed. Given the circumstances, he's unable to carry out the intervention and, therefore, can't meet his expected outcome.

Reassess the patient's condition to determine whether the intervention you performed (assisting the patient to dangle his legs before standing) caused the response (dizziness, tachycardia, and hypotension) or whether the response is a sign or symptom of a worsening condition or a complication. Ask yourself the following questions:

- Is this response a continuation or exacerbation of an existing problem or condition?
- Is this response due to something that has changed in the patient's condition?
- Is this a new problem that needs to be addressed by a revision of the care plan?

Subtle signs

During evaluation, always pay attention to even slight changes in assessment findings. Sometimes, a mild physiological adaptation, such as a response to a position change, can mimic a subtle change in condition. Because of a relative lack of clinical experience, student nurses commonly have difficulty making such distinctions, which can affect the care plans they create for patients. Remember, when you're in doubt, you and your patient will benefit most if you ask for help from another nurse or from your instructor.

The power of reassessment

When evaluation reveals changes in a patient's condition or expected outcomes that haven't been achieved by the nursing interventions set out in the care plan or when your interventions create an unexpected patient response that leads to new symptoms or a worsening of the patient's condition, you must reassess not only the patient but also your expectations for the patient (expected outcome). In some cases, the care plan will need to be revised to reflect a different patient outcome and a new set of interventions.

Short-term goals are those that can be accomplished during the patient's hospital stay, usually within a week.

Documenting changes

Remember to document (electronic or handwritten) the patient's changed condition. Use the format preferred by your facility for this documentation. Also document any calls that you make that informs the practitioner (physician or nurse practitioner) of changes in the patient's condition, including the time and date the call was made.

Writing evaluation statements

Part of the evaluation process involves writing a statement that describes whether the patient has achieved the expected outcome (short- or long-term goal) as it was written into the care plan.

Revisiting goals

As you may recall, short-term goals are those that can be accomplished during the patient's hospital stay (usually within 1 week or less), whereas long-term goals are those that can be accomplished over an extended time (usually more than 1 week).

May I opine?

Your evaluation statement should indicate whether the expected outcome was achieved. However, your documentation just prior to the evaluation statement should list the evidence supporting this conclusion. This evidence is the information you obtained in your reassessment and evaluation. These conclusions can state that an outcome has been fully met, partially met, or not met.

Write right

In your documentation, your evaluation should contain three types of information:
- results of your reassessment
- results of your comparison of the reassessment data with the patient's baseline data or normal findings

- evaluation statement that specifies the patient's status toward achieving the expected outcomes.

Evaluating short-term goals

Your evaluation of a short-term goal should occur within the time frame established in the patient outcome statement. You should determine the patient's progress toward achieving the goal within the time frame and revise the care plan if needed. Keep in mind that your patient may have more than one short-term goal for each nursing diagnosis.

Let's walk through it together

For example, if a patient outcome states that "The patient will ambulate in the hallway two times with minimal assistance on the evening shift on 6/22/17," you must evaluate the patient's progress toward accomplishing that goal by the end of your shift on that day. If the patient fails to achieve the goal by the end of your shift, you must document this in the medical record in the form of an evaluation statement, such as "Patient was unable to tolerate second attempt at ambulating in hallway with assistance; expected outcome not met." Of course, your reassessment data supporting this evaluation would be documented in the medical record according to the format used in the facility.

Long-term goals take more time to accomplish— sometimes weeks or months.

Evaluating long-term goals

Your patient's long-term goal may be the desired end result of nursing care or, in some cases, a goal that extends beyond the usual time frame of his or her hospital stay. Such conditions as stroke, myocardial infarction, traumatic brain injury, neurologic or spinal injury, hip fracture, and Alzheimer's disease commonly require long-term goals that extend over a continuum of care. Typically, patients with these conditions are discharged from the hospital to a long-term care facility or home health agency for continued nursing treatment and care.

Taking the long road home

For example, the patient with a nursing diagnosis of *Toileting self-care deficit related to weakness as evidenced by muscle strength 4/6 in lower extremities, a prior order for bed rest, and loss of muscle mass due to aging* may have the following expected outcome: "Ambulate to bathroom with minimal assistance within 1 month after discharge to nursing rehabilitation center."

Such a goal establishes a clear timeline for evaluating the outcome (within 1 month) and sets the criteria (with assistance, after discharge from the hospital or transfer to the rehabilitation center).

Evaluating the care plan

In addition to periodically evaluating the patient's status and progress toward achieving outcomes, you'll need to evaluate the care plan in its entirety. This means going through each section of the plan to determine whether the patient's problems have been resolved, outcomes have been achieved, and interventions are still appropriate and current.

Reevaluating the care plan is just as important as reevaluating the patient.

Reviewing the plan

Your reassessment of the care plan will yield much information about what you and the patient have accomplished and what care still needs to be done. Ask yourself the following questions, taking each section in turn.

Look at the nursing diagnoses

- Does the patient still have the same problems (nursing diagnoses)? If so, has the focus of any of the problems changed in a way that would warrant rewriting the diagnosis?
- Were the diagnoses confirmed or ruled out?
- Does the patient have any new needs? If so, should any additional diagnoses be added to the care plan?
- Are all of the diagnoses prioritized?

Check patient outcomes

- Has the patient achieved the short- and long-term outcomes for each nursing diagnosis?
- Is each goal still valid and achievable within its given time frame?
- Should the care plan include any additional criteria for achieving the outcomes?
- Does the patient agree with the stated outcomes?
- If the patient didn't achieve the outcomes, do you know why?

Review the interventions

- Do the interventions address the patient's specific needs?
- Are they achievable within the designated time frames?
- Are they clearly written so that other team members can follow them?
- Should any interventions be discontinued or rewritten?

Evaluating the plan

Once you've reviewed the care plan, you can provide a written evaluation (on the care plan itself or in your progress notes) of each expected outcome of the patient. Be sure to base your evaluation on information gathered from all sources, including your own observations and findings, the patient's medical record, the patient himself, the patient's family, and other members of the health care team.

Record your evaluation using standard terminology that all team members can easily understand and follow. For example, use the following words:

- *Continue:* No change in diagnosis, patient outcomes, or interventions is needed at this time, and the diagnosis hasn't yet been resolved.
- *Revised:* No change in diagnosis is needed, but the patient's expected outcomes and the associated interventions have been updated to reflect the patient's current status.
- *Discontinued:* A change in diagnosis is needed because additional data collection has shown that the diagnosis is no longer appropriate for the patient.
- *Achieved:* All expected outcomes have been met and the diagnosis is no longer appropriate for the patient, or one expected outcome has been met and, therefore, that portion of the care plan is marked "achieved" while the other outcomes are ongoing.
- *Reinstate:* A previous diagnosis whose outcomes had all been achieved requires renewal because the problem has recurred.

Updating the care plan

In some cases, you'll need to make modifications to the patient's care plan as a result of your evaluation. Updating typically begins with determining whether the patient has achieved the outcomes. If the outcomes haven't been fully met but your assessment shows that the problem is resolved or was inappropriately identified, the plan can be discontinued. If the problem persists, continue the plan with new outcome target dates until the desired status is achieved. If the outcomes are partially met or unmet, identify interfering factors, such as misinterpreted information or a change in the patient's status, and revise the outcomes and interventions accordingly.

When plan A doesn't work...

Updating may involve:
- clarifying or amending the database to reflect new information
- reexamining and correcting nursing diagnoses
- establishing outcome criteria that reflect new information and new or amended nursing strategies

- adding the revised nursing care plan to the original document
- recording the rationale for the revision in the progress notes.

...go to plan B...

For instance, in the case of the patient who couldn't tolerate getting out of bed to use the bathroom, even with assistance (see page 150), you could change the nursing diagnosis, patient outcome, and interventions based on the inferences you made when comparing the baseline patient data with his reassessment findings. (See *Updating a care plan.*)

...or plan C

In the event that the patient can't tolerate the activities associated with sitting on the side of the bed and, therefore, can't meet the outcome goal, revise the care plan again, beginning with your reassessment. Other nursing diagnoses that can be established based on the given findings and reassessment data may include:

- *Deficient fluid volume*
- *Risk for injury.*

Keeping priorities straight

Be sure to reprioritize the nursing diagnoses when updating your care plan. This is especially important when the patient experiences unexpected changes in condition or possibly untoward reactions as a result of his treatment or care.

When reprioritizing diagnoses, ask yourself these questions:

- Will the patient's progress be hindered if the problem isn't managed now?
- Will the patient lose functional status if the problem isn't managed now?
- Will the patient be harmed in any way that will produce a detrimental outcome if the problem isn't managed now?

A new outcome

If you're changing the nursing diagnoses, follow through by updating the expected patient outcomes (remember to include realistic, measurable goals) and specific interventions needed to achieve them. Also, make sure your interventions address any new treatments or required care (independent or interprofessional) resulting from the patient's changed condition.

Last but not least

Document all of your evaluations and, as a student nurse, communicate your findings to your instructor and the patient's primary care nurse. Be sure to follow the facility's procedure for documentation and update of nursing care plans.

Memory jogger

If you know you need to revise your patient's care plan but can't remember where to start, think

Redo:

Reassess the patient.

Evaluate your findings.

Decide on a course of action.

Organize the care plan accordingly.

Updating a care plan

After your 78-year-old patient's experience with attempting to dangle and stand upright before walking into the bathroom, you reevaluate the established care plan. After careful reassessment, you update his care plan to include an additional nursing diagnosis and expected outcomes. One possible update is presented below:

Date	Nursing diagnosis	Expected outcomes	Interventions	Outcome evaluation (initials and date)
4/1/17	Activity intolerance related to aging process and hypovolemia as evidenced by weakness, dizziness, and increased pulse rate during activity	The patient will tolerate sitting up at the side of the bed with assistance for 10 minutes, twice per day on 7‼3 shift.	• Assess *functional level* every shift as needed. • *Obtain positional vital signs,* oxygen saturation level, and pain level before starting any activity and compare these findings with morning baseline data. • Assess patient intake and output over the past 24 hours. • *Monitor for signs of* fatigue and avoid activity during this period. • *Maintain the patient's* safety. • *Raise the head of the bed* incrementally to reduce dizziness. • *Help the patient sit on* the side of the bed with the assistance of two support personnel. • *Remain with the patient* the entire time he's sitting upright, and assess for changes in condition or activity intolerance. • *Report significant changes* in the patient's condition or activity intolerance to the practitioner.	

REVIEW DATES		
Date	**Signature**	**Initials**
4/1/17	Amanda Trotter	AT

On the case

Case study background

You're assigned to care for Ella Racer, a 70-year-old admitted 3 days ago with dehydration. In reviewing the admission assessment data, you note that admission vital signs were blood pressure 90/50 mm Hg, heart rate 110 beats/minute, and respiratory rate 18 breaths/minute. Her skin color was pale, and skin turgor was poor. Her weight is 145 lb (usual weight 151 lb). Initial laboratory studies indicated an elevated serum sodium level and serum osmolarity. Her care plan includes the nursing diagnosis *Deficient fluid volume related to active loss through diarrhea and inadequate intake.* Her expected outcomes are:

- The patient's fluid volume will return to normal and remain normal as evidenced by stable vital signs and a urine output at the volume established for the patient by day 3 of hospitalization.
- The patient's electrolyte values will stay within a normal range by discharge.
- The patient will express and identify three ways to prevent dehydration by discharge.
  Nursing interventions for this patient include:
- Monitor and record vital signs every 2 hours.
- Measure and record intake and output every hour. Report a urine output less than 30 mL/hour.
- Administer fluids as ordered and monitor and record effectiveness of therapy.
- Administer antidiarrheal medication as ordered.
- Weigh the patient daily at the same time.
- Monitor electrolyte levels and report abnormal values.
- Explain reasons for fluid loss and teach the patient how to avoid further episodes.

Your reassessment on day 3 reveals the following vital signs: blood pressure 110/60 mm Hg, heart rate 75 beats/minute, and respiratory rate 16 breaths/minute. Urine output is greater than 30 mL/hour. Dextrose 5% in water is infusing IV at 50 mL/hour. Skin color is pink, and skin turgor is normal. The patient has experienced no further episodes of diarrhea and is tolerating oral fluids and solids. Electrolyte levels are within normal limits. The patient states, "I don't know how I can prevent this from happening again."

Critical thinking exercise

1. What reassessment findings show that the interventions are working?

   _____
   _____
   _____
   _____
   _____
   _____

2. Which interventions may no longer be necessary or could be altered?

_____

_____

_____

_____

_____

_____

3. Which of the patient's short-term goals hasn't been met?

_____

_____

_____

_____

_____

_____

Answer key

Critical thinking exercise

1. Reassessment findings that show that interventions are working include vital signs that have returned to within normal limits (blood pressure 110/60 mm Hg, heart rate 75 beats/minute, and respiratory rate 16 breaths/minute); urine output greater than 30 mL/hour; normal skin turgor; oral fluid toleration; and electrolyte levels within normal limits.
2. Because the patient is now stable, vital signs no longer need to be taken every 2 hours. Monitoring every 4 hours or 8 hours would be adequate. Urine output could also now be measured every 4 to 8 hours.
3. Because the patient stated "I don't know how I can prevent this from happening again," the goal of "The patient will express and identify three ways to prevent dehydration by discharge" hasn't been met.

Selected references

Alfaro-LeFevre, R. (2014). *Applying nursing process*. Philadelphia, PA: Wolter Kluwer.

American Nurse Association. (2015). *Nursing scope and standards of performance and standards of clinical practice* (3rd ed.). Silver Spring, MD: nursesbooks.org.

Hinkle, J., & Cheever, K. (2014). *Brunner & Suddarth's textbook of medical-surgical nursing* (13th ed). New York, NY: Lippincott Williams & Wilkins.

2017 National Patient Safety Goals: https://www.jointcommission.org/standards_information/npsgs.aspx

Nettina, S. (2014). *Lippincott's manual of nursing practice* (10th ed.). New York, NY: Lippincott Williams & Wilkins.

Taylor, C., & Lillis, P. (2014). *Fundamentals of nursing; The art and science of person-centered nursing care* (8th ed.). Philadelphia, PA: Lippincott Williams & Wilkins.

Chapter 7

Putting it all together

Just the facts

In this chapter, you'll learn:

♦ techniques for using traditional and standardized care plans

♦ the role of computers in generating care plans

♦ components of and uses for a critical pathway

♦ types of care plans used in different health care settings.

Another look at the nursing care plan

By now, you're probably fairly well versed in the nursing process and its relationship to the nursing care plan. You know the five steps of the nursing process—assessment, nursing diagnosis, planning, implementation, and evaluation—and understand that each step builds on the previous one and that all the steps interconnect, forming the basis of a care plan.

But how does it all come together? How do you gather all the necessary information about a patient and document it correctly? And where do you, as a nursing student, fit in?

Why you need a care plan

The nursing care plan is the core of your nursing practice—a vital source of information about your patient's problems, needs, and goals and the quintessential blueprint to direct your treatment and care. When well executed, this document can lead you step-by-step through your busy workday and help put your patient squarely on the road to wellness.

Flexible, but permanent record

Until 1991, a care plan wasn't a required part of a patient's permanent record. It may have been used by the nursing staff but, in some facilities, it was discarded when a patient was discharged. Now, the Joint Commission mandates that the nursing care plan be permanently

This chapter will help you put together the pieces of the care planning process.

Weighing the evidence

When did the Joint Commission become "The Boss"?

The Joint Commission (Joint Commission on Accreditation of Healthcare Organizations [JCAHO]) is often cited as the authority on standards of practice within health care organizations. However, the Joint Commission itself doesn't claim to originate standards of practice. By incorporating them into the accreditation process, the Joint Commission promotes compliance with those standards that the members of a profession have deemed essential for best practice within their specialty. This can mean engineering standards for building safety or nursing standards for excellence in provision of nursing care. The American Nurses Association and related specialty nursing organizations have determined that the nursing process, as embodied in an individualized patient care plan, is the standard of care expected of a nurse.

integrated into the medical record by paper or electronic means. (See *When did the Joint Commission become "The Boss"?*)

Joint Commission policy changes have also led to greater flexibility when writing care plans. The commission no longer specifies the format for documenting patient care, so new methods have emerged that can make planning faster and easier.

By nurses, but not just for nurses

Nursing is a unique patient-focused profession that's different from medicine and other health care fields, having its own set of diagnoses and outcomes and interventions that can be customized to meet each patient's needs. However, nurses don't work in a vacuum; they work in collaboration with other interprofessional team members to promote patient health and wellness. Consequently, although nursing care plans are developed by nurses, they may be used as a springboard to a team plan by the entire interprofessional team, including:

- nurses (clinical nurse specialists, registered nurses, licensed practical nurses, and nursing students)
- practitioners (physicians, physician's assistants, nurse practitioners, and midwives)
- physical and occupational therapists
- speech-language pathologists
- dietitians

The expanding world of care planning

The nursing profession isn't the only profession concerned with demonstrating the unique and crucial nature of their skills in the health care setting. Like nurses, other health care providers are seeking ways to show that their actions reflect professional accountability and represent reimbursable services from insurance companies.

Respiratory, physical, and occupational therapists; registered dietitians; speech-language pathologists; and nutritional specialists all assess patients, analyze their findings, develop treatment plans, implement their plans, and reassess the effectiveness of their plans. The standards of practice for these professionals make it clear that these are mandated functions.

In many long-term care facilities, assisted-living facilities, inpatient psychiatric centers, and home care and hospice agencies, these professionals are active members of an interprofessional team that develops an overall care plan for each patient. As such, a dietitian might collaborate with nursing staff to include specific interventions in the nursing care plan that promote certain outcomes—for example, obtaining optimal nutrition for skin integrity. A physical or occupational therapist might be involved in developing some of the nursing interventions for a patient with a diagnosis of *Impaired physical mobility*. Depending on the facility, these specialists may document their assessment findings and care on an interprofessional form or their own standard forms.

- respiratory therapists
- social workers and discharge planners
- pharmacists
- clergy.

All on the same team

Each member of the interprofessional team may have some input in developing the care plan, but the registered nurse is responsible for making sure that it's carried out on a daily basis and documented according to the facility's policies. Other team members can also document their interventions on the care plan under their specified column or box. (See *The expanding world of care planning*.)

Students' role in care planning

As a student, you should read and be knowledgeable about your patient's care plan at the hospital, nursing home, or agency where you perform clinical rounds. Each facility and department operates

Teacher knows best

Paper trail

As you proceed through your clinical rotations, the type of paperwork you're required to complete might change. An early focus may be on the nursing assessment and correlating those findings with the medical history and diagnosis. Later, you may be required to complete medication work sheets that focus on helping you learn about hundreds of drugs and what to teach the patients taking them. Finally come the nursing care plans themselves, in various formats and detail. All of these tools serve one essential purpose: to broaden your knowledge base and sharpen your critical thinking skills so you can make decisions logically and quickly as you care for patients.

differently, so it's your responsibility to become familiar with the system used.

RN recording rights

Keep in mind that only registered nurses can create and update a nursing care plan. In some institutions, licensed practical nurses can assist with writing the care plan, but they're only permitted to do so under the supervision of a registered nurse. The registered nurse remains the one accountable for accurate collection of patient data, development of a problem list and pertinent nursing diagnoses, devising appropriate expected outcomes for the patient and corresponding nursing interventions, implementing the plan of care, and evaluating the plan. The registered professional nurse is the only team member permitted to change the nursing portions of the plan.

Student's right to write

As a student, you may use and follow the established care plan, but you can't document on it. However, you're expected to create your own care plan or concept map to use during clinical rotations. Even when you don't have to turn in a written care plan to your instructor, you're accountable for having developed a care plan for the day and being able to verbalize it to your instructor when asked. (See *Paper trail*.)

Types of care plans

Care plans are usually written in one of two styles: traditional or standardized. As a student or a newly graduated nurse, you're more likely to see and use standardized care plans; in most cases, they're easier to use and they're more common than traditional plans. Another issue is the increasing use of electronic health records systems that include a care planning function. These systems are a variation on standardized care plans but require some special mention. Regardless of which type you use, your care plan should cover all aspects of nursing care, from admission to discharge.

Traditional care plans

Also called an *individually developed plan,* a traditional care plan is written to your patient's specific problems and causative factors. After you analyze your assessment data for a patient, you either write the plan by hand or enter it into a computer. (See *Traditional, but highly personalized,* page 158.)

Home-baked from scratch

The basic form for the traditional care plan varies, depending on the function of this important document in your facility or department. Most forms have four main columns:
1. nursing diagnoses
2. expected outcomes
3. interventions
4. outcome evaluations.
   The form may also have columns for the date when you initiated the care plan, target dates for expected outcomes, and the dates for review, revisions, and resolutions. Most forms also have a place for you to sign or initial whenever you make an entry or revision.

Traditional care plans can be written by hand or entered into a computer.

Looking toward an outcome

The information that you should include on a traditional care plan form varies, too. Because shorter hospital stays are more common today, in some facilities, you're expected to write only short-term outcomes that the patient can reach by the time he's discharged. However, other facilities—especially long-term care facilities—may also want you to chart long-term outcomes for the patient's maximum functioning level. These facilities commonly provide forms with separate spaces for short-term and long-term outcomes.

Personal, visual, clear

The traditional method has several advantages:
- It provides a personalized plan for each patient.
- The format allows health care team members and the patient to easily visualize the plan.
- Columns for outcome evaluations are clearly delineated.

Traditional, but highly personalized

Here's an example of a traditional care plan. It shows how these forms are typically organized. Remember that a traditional plan is written from scratch for each patient. These types of plans are becoming less common with the advent of electronic products containing modifiable standardized care plans.

Date	Nursing diagnosis	Interventions	Outcome evaluation (initials and date)
6/27/17	Ineffective breathing Pattern R/T alteration in depth of breathing due to pain as evidenced by patient report of pain with deep breaths or coughing and shallow respirations at 22 to 24 breaths/minute	• Assess and record respiration status, including pulse oximetry q4h at 12–4–8. • Note use of accessory muscles, nasal flaring, irritability, confusion, or lethargy. • Observe for signs of cyanosis. • Assess for pain q3h and 1 hour after each dosage of medication. • Give pain medication as ordered. • Assist patient to upright or semi-Fowler's position q2h while awake on even hours. • Teach patient how, when, and why to use incentive spirometer. • Demonstrate to patient how to splint chest while coughing. • Encourage patient to use spirometer 10 times/hour while awake as long as bed rest is maintained. • Assist the patient with walking 3 times/day. • Initiate oxygen therapy as ordered per given parameters.	

Time isn't on its side

The main disadvantage of a traditional plan is that it's time-consuming to read and write because it requires lengthy documentation.

Standardized care plans

Standardized care plans are more commonly used. They eliminate the problems associated with traditional plans by using preprinted information. This saves documentation time. (See *Standardized saves time*, page 160.)

Some standardized plans are classified by medical diagnoses or diagnosis-related groups (DRGs); others, by nursing diagnoses. The preprinted information included in a standardized care plan includes interventions for patients with similar diagnoses and, usually, root outcome statements.

Insist on individuality

Early versions of standardized care plans didn't allow for differences in patients' needs. However, current versions require you to explain how you have individualized the plan for each patient by adding the following information:

Standardized care plans are commonly completed on a computer.

- "related to" (R/T) statements and signs and symptoms for a nursing diagnosis—If the form provides a root diagnosis, such as "Acute pain R/T," you might fill in *inflammation, as exhibited by grimacing and other expressions of pain.*
- time limits for the outcomes—To a root statement of the goal *Perform postural drainage without assistance,* you might add *for 15 minutes immediately on awakening in the morning by 11/17.*
- frequency of interventions—To an intervention such as *Perform passive range-of-motion exercises,* you might add *twice per day: in the morning and in the evening.*
- specific instruction for interventions—For the standard intervention *Elevate the patient's head,* you might specify *before sleep, on three pillows.*

Computers make combos less cumbersome

When a patient has more than one diagnosis, you must use all the standardized care plans, which can make records long and cumbersome. However, if your facility uses computerized standardized care plans, you may be able to extract only the parts you need for each plan and then combine them to make one manageable plan. Some computer programs provide a checklist of interventions from which you can select to build your own plans.

Although standardized plans usually include only essential information, most provide space for you to write additional expected outcomes, interventions, and outcome evaluations.

Standardized saves time

A standardized care plan can save you valuable time. The plan below is for a patient with a nursing diagnosis of *Impaired tissue integrity*. To customize this standardized care plan to one of your patients, you would complete the diagnosis—including signs and symptoms—and fill in the expected outcomes.

Date *4/15/17*	**Nursing diagnosis** **Impaired tissue integrity** *Related to peripheral arterial disease evidenced by pain and stage 2 pressure ulcer on ℝ fourth toe, sluggish capillary refill in right foot, and cool temperature of right foot compared to left.*
Target date	**Expected outcomes**
4/17/17	Attains relief from symptoms: *Pain will resolve.*
4/17/17	Verbalizes intent to abstain from aggravating behavior: *Patient wears nicotine patch and intends to stop smoking.*
4/17/17	Maintains collateral circulation: *Bilateral + 1 peripheral pulses in lower extremities are palpable.*
4/17/17	Verbalizes intent to follow specific management routine after discharge: *Patient describes the foot care regimen and physical therapy exercises recommended.*
Date *4/15/17*	**Interventions** Assess skin/tissue integrity q6h at 0200-0800-1400-2000 (military time). Provide foot and ulcer care. Administer and monitor treatments according to facility protocols. Maintain adequate hydration. Monitor I/O: *q8h* Elevate the head of bed to: *45 to 60°* Encourage adherence to an exercise regimen as tolerated. Educate the patient about risk factors and injury prevention measures. Refer the patient to a stop-smoking program on discharge. Additional interventions: *Assess peripheral pulses, skin temperature and color, and capillary refill q6h at 0200-0800-1400-2000. Administer analgesics before ulcer care and physical therapy as ordered prn.*
Date	**Outcome evaluation**
4/17/17	Attained relief of immediate symptoms: *Pain and edema resolved, stage 2 ulcer continues; outcome partially met, extend expected outcome to 4/19/17 or discharge if earlier.*
4/17/17	
4/17/17	Maintained collateral circulation: *Palpable peripheral pulses bilaterally, right diminished compared to left; right lower extremity cooler to touch than left; capillary refill sluggish but equal bilaterally; outcome partially met, extend expected outcome to 4/19/17 or discharge if earlier.*
4/17/17	Verbalized intent to follow specific management routines after discharge: *Patient can describe foot care and exercise guidelines; outcome met.*

The pros

Standardized care plans offer many advantages because they:
- require far less writing than traditional plans
- are more legible
- are easier to duplicate
- make compliance with a facility's policy easier for all members of the health care team, including experts, novices, and ancillary staff
- guide you in creating the plan and allow you the freedom to adapt it to your patient.

The cons (there's always at least one)

This method has one main drawback: If you simply check off items on a list or fill in the blanks, you might not individualize the patient's care or document your findings adequately.

Computerized care plans

In the health care industry, the first area of extensive conversion to electronics was institutional accounting. However, in the past 15 years, the push has been toward integrating accounting systems with a complete electronic health record (EHR). Today, you're increasingly likely to encounter computerized care plans during your clinical rotations.

Different strokes for different folks

Various types of software are available for different facility needs. Some systems are programmed to generate a list of nursing diagnoses after the patient's assessment data are entered. You can modify the selected items as needed. Others require you to choose the diagnoses yourself from a master list. The system then adds these diagnoses to the patient's EHR.

EHRs also offer different styles of care planning. Some systems rely on generalized care plans written to a patient problem or profile, not to a specific nursing diagnosis. For example, in the sample electronic shift report shown on pages 120 to 122, note that the patient's care plan was called "General care of the adult" and included two nursing protocols (Falls prevention and Skin breakdown [prevention]), plus a clinical guideline. A very general goal is listed: "Patient will tolerate a progressive increase in activity level." However, some EHR products are moving toward integrating the taxonomies of NANDA International, Nursing Interventions Classification, and Nursing Outcomes Classification into the process.

RN input

Like traditional and standardized plans, a computerized care plan must be reviewed by a registered nurse every 24 hours. Remember that despite their efficiency and ability to access information quickly, computer software systems can't replace a nurse's critical thinking and decision-making skills. Nurses still have to decide which diagnoses and interventions are most appropriate for any given patient and must evaluate when changes to the care plan are needed.

Care plans in different settings

As you begin your clinical rotations, you'll notice that different units and care settings sometimes use different care plan formats. For example, acute care units, including psychiatric centers, commonly use standardized care plans or critical pathways. Same-day surgery units often use a problem list format rather than an actual care plan, but it serves the same purpose.

Note that different care settings use different types of care plans.

Have diagnosis, will travel

The standardized care plans available on each unit are usually selected to fit the type of patient medical diagnoses common to the unit. For example, a medical-surgical unit might have different standard plans than the maternity or psychiatric unit. However, a resource containing all plans should be available to all staff because patients may have more than one diagnosis, some of which may not be included in the standardized plans for the patient's assigned unit. For example, a patient on a psychiatric unit may have coexisting nursing diagnoses related to an ongoing medical diagnosis, such as diabetes or gastro-esophageal reflux disease. Conversely, a patient with schizophrenia may be admitted to an oncology unit for treatment of cancer. Holistic patient care requires attention to all diagnoses because each impacts the patient's healing capacity.

Acute care hospital units

On most acute care units, care plans are separate documents that are formulated at the time of a patient's admission (typically within the first 8 to 12 hours). Although nursing interventions begin immediately with a patient's admission, the care plan takes careful planning and collaborative input and serves as a legal document of the care being given.

Most facilities require that care plans be reviewed and updated by a registered nurse at least every 24 hours, beginning with the time of admission. Accreditation organizations, such as the Joint Commission, perform spot checks of individual patient charts to see whether a care plan is present and if it was reviewed within the established time frame.

Fill in the blanks…

Some units use preprinted plans on which the nursing diagnosis is already written; the nurse fills in a "related to" clause as well as individualized interventions, making the care plan specific to the patient. For example, for a patient with a nursing diagnosis of *Acute pain*, the nurse might fill in *related to surgical procedure*, depending on the reason for the pain. The interventions, of course, would be filled in based on the patient's needs and circumstances.

…or check 'em off

Other units use preprinted care plans that include a comprehensive list of interventions. In this case, the nurse simply checks off the interventions applicable to the patient's problem.

Multiple problems

Usually, patients on medical-surgical units have multiple nursing diagnoses that must be addressed. All of the diagnoses for one patient are considered one care plan. For example, a patient admitted with a fractured left tibia might have the following diagnoses:
- *Acute pain related to compound fracture of tibia*
- *Risk for infection related to multiple breaks in skin integrity of left leg*
- *Impaired physical mobility related to fractured left tibia as evidenced by inability to bear weight on left leg and X-rays showing compound fracture.*

Keeping priorities straight

Within the care plan, the nursing diagnoses must be prioritized according to the level of importance for the patient. For example, suppose you've assessed a patient admitted with acute heart failure and have identified these diagnoses:
- *Excess fluid volume related to sodium and water retention*
- *Activity intolerance related to shortness of breath and fatigue*
- *Decreased cardiac output related to impaired contractility*
- *Impaired urinary elimination (hesitancy) related to benign prostate enlargement*
- *Ineffective peripheral tissue perfusion related to decreased cardiac output*

- *Anxiety related to acute increase in shortness of breath.*
  You might *prioritize* these nursing diagnoses as follows:
- *Decreased cardiac output related to impaired contractility*
- *Excess fluid volume related to sodium and water retention*
- *Ineffective tissue perfusion related to decreased cardiac output*
- *Anxiety related to acute increase in shortness of breath.*
- *Impaired urinary elimination(hesitancy) related to benign prostate enlargement*
- *Activity intolerance related to shortness of breath and fatigue*

Take the critical pathway

A critical pathway is a special type of care plan that's used by the interprofessional team, not just nurses, so it's more collaborative in nature. It includes assessment criteria, interventions, treatments, and outcomes for specific conditions according to a timeline that's based on an average patient's expected length of stay. Actual time frames can be modified to meet each patient's needs.

Complete coverage

Think of a critical pathway as a predetermined checklist describing the tasks you and the patient must accomplish. Unlike a nursing care plan, it has an interprofessional focus, covering all of the patient's problems, not just those identified during a nursing assessment. For example, it may include specific interventions for physical assessment, lab work and procedures, consultations, medication administration, nutrition, elimination, activity and therapy, patient teaching, and discharge planning. (See *Using a critical pathway,* pages 166 to 167.)

Think of a critical pathway as a predetermined checklist that describes the steps you and the patient must take.

Same-day surgery unit

On a same-day surgery unit, nurses may follow an abbreviated standardized plan that addresses the patient's specific type of surgery or procedure. Additional medical diagnoses are listed and interventions are added related to those diagnoses if needed. The nurse typically reviews the problem list before and after the surgery or procedure. If the patient requires admittance to the hospital, a full nursing care plan is developed, using the problem list as a starting point.

Extended-care facilities

Nursing homes and other extended-care facilities have a different system for formulating care plans. Most of these facilities provide services for individuals who qualify for Medicare or Medicaid insurance benefits due to their age or severe disability. Medicare regulations have become the standard of care for extended-care facilities so that even private insurers look for verification that a facility meets these standards. Part of these standards requires the completion of the Minimum Data Set (MDS) form, which documents patient assessment and care screening and guides reimbursement levels. Each facility employs a registered nurse as the RN Assessment Coordinator (RNAC). This person is responsible for completing and submitting the MDS and other required forms and running the weekly interprofessional team meetings at which care plans are finalized and reviewed for each resident. The RNAC meets with residents and their families, communicates with all staff members involved in the resident's care, and reviews all documentation to verify that required information has been completed.

Mirror, mirror on the wall

If you have a chance to do a clinical rotation in an extended-care facility, you may find that this setting most closely mirrors the use of the nursing process and nursing and interprofessional care planning as you have been taught in school. Because residents have chronic conditions requiring 24-hour care, nursing diagnoses may be relevant for long periods. Expected outcomes tend to focus less on healing and resumption of prior function than on maintaining the present level of function and developing skills to adapt to limitations in function. However, always be alert for those situations in which a rehabilitative goal is appropriate, such as fractured bones, episodic lung or urinary tract infections, situational depression or anxiety disorders, or new urinary incontinence issues.

Don't break the rules

An RNAC has up to 7 days to complete the MDS and 14 days to develop an individualized care plan for each new resident. In the meantime, a generic care plan must be initiated within 24 hours. Common nursing diagnoses in extended-care facilities include:
- *Chronic pain*
- *Risk for injury*
- *Risk for fall*
- *Activity intolerance*
- *Risk for infection*
- *Risk for impaired skin integrity*
- *Impaired environmental interpretation syndrome.*

Each resident must have a complete reassessment yearly, including a complete physical examination by a physician. Guidelines have been set for frequency of documentation by each discipline, review of the medical orders, and evaluation and updating of the interprofessional care plan.

(Text continues on page 168.)

Using a critical pathway

At any point in a patient's treatment, a glance at the critical pathway allows you to compare the patient's progress and your performance as a caregiver with the usual course of care and progress for other patients with the same diagnosis. Critical pathways are based on analytical studies as well as the standards of care established by the professional group most closely allied with treatment of the disorder.

Example

The standard critical pathway below outlines care for a patient with a colon resection.

CRITICAL PATHWAY: COLON RESECTION WITHOUT COLOSTOMY				
	Patient visit	Presurgery day 1	Day 0 O.R. day	Postoperative day 1
Assessments	History and physical with breast, rectal, and pelvic examinations Nursing assessment	Nursing admission assessment	Nursing admission assessment on TBA patients in holding area Postoperative review of systems assessment*	Review of systems assessment*
Consults	Social service consult Physical therapy consult	Notify referring doctor of impending admission		
Labs and diagnostics	Complete blood count (CBC) PT/PTT Electrocardiogram Chest X-ray (CXR) Chemistry profile CT scan ABD w/wo contrast CT scan pelvis Urinalysis Barium enema and flexible sigmoidoscopy or colonoscopy Biopsy report	Type and screen for patients with Hgb level less than 10	Type and screen for patients in holding area with Hgb level less than 10	CBC
Interventions	Many or all of the above labs and diagnostics will have already been done. Check all results and fax to the surgeon's office.	Admit by 0800. Check for bowel preparation orders \n\n Bowel preparation* Antiembolism stockings Incentive spirometry Ankle exercises* IV access* Routine VS* Pneumatic inflation boots	Shave and prepare in operating room. NG tube maintenance* I/O VS per routine* Foley care* Incentive spirometry* Ankle exercises* IV site care* HOB 30° Safety measures Wound care* Mouth care*	NG tube maintenance* I/O* VS per routine* Foley care* Incentive spirometry* Ankle exercises* IV site care* HOB 30°* Safety measures* Wound care* Mouth care* Antiembolism stockings
IVs		IV fluids, D5 ½ NSS	IV fluids, D_5LR	I.V
Medication	Prescribe GoLYTELY or NuLYTELY at 1000 and 1400. Neomycin at 0800, 1500, and 2200 Erythromycin at 0800, 1500, and 2200	GoLYTELY or NuLYTELY at 1000 and 1400 Erythromycin at 0800, 1500, and 2200 Neomycin at 0800, 1500, and 2200	Preoperative ABX in holding area Postoperative ABX _ 2 doses PCA (basal rate 0.5 mg) subQ heparin	P S
Diet/GI	Clear liquids presurgery day. NPO after midnight	Clear liquids presurgery day. NPO after midnight	NPO/NG tube	
Activity			4 hours after surgery, ambulate with abdominal binder.* D/C pneumatic inflation boots after patient ambulates	Ambulate t.i.d. with abdominal binder.* May shower Physical therapy b.i.d.
KEY: * = NSG **Activities** V = Variance N = No variance \n\n **Signatures:**	1. 2. 3. \n V V V \n Ⓝ N N \n\n 1. C. Molloy, RN 2. ____ 3. ____	1. 2. 3. \n V V V \n Ⓝ Ⓝ Ⓝ \n\n 1. M Connel, RN 2. J. Smith, RN 3. P. Joseph, RN	1. 2. 3. \n V V V \n Ⓝ Ⓝ Ⓝ \n\n 1. L. Singer, RN 2. J. Smith, RN 3. P. Joseph, RN	1. 2. 3. \n V V V \n Ⓝ Ⓝ Ⓝ \n\n 1. L. Singer, RN 2. J. Smith, RN 3. P. Joseph, RN

The pathway designates a specific time frame for patient care activities.

The pathway is organized into categories based on the patient's medical diagnosis.

The pathway lists tasks that the patient and caregivers need to accomplish.

CRITICAL PATHWAY: COLON RESECTION WITHOUT COLOSTOMY

	Postoperative day 2	Postoperative day 3	Postoperative day 4	Postoperative day 5
Assessments	Review of systems assessment*	Review of systems assessment*	Review of systems assessment*	Review of systems assessment*
Consults		Dietary consult		Oncology consult if indicated (Dukes B2 or C or high-risk lesion) (or to be done as outpatient)
Labs and diagnostics	Electrolyte 7 (EL-7) CXR	CBC EL-7	Pathology results on chart	CBC EL-7
Interventions	Discontinue NG tube if possible* (per guidelines). I/O* VS per routine* Discontinue Foley* Ambulating* Incentive spirometry* Ankle exercises* IV site care* HOB 30°* Safety measures* Wound care* Mouth care* Antiembolism stockings	I/O* VS per routine* Incentive spirometry* Ankle exercises* IV site care* Safety measures* Wound care* Antiembolism stockings	I/O* VS per routine* Incentive spirometry* Ankle exercises* IV site care* Safety measures* Wound care* Antiembolism stockings	Consider staple removal Replace with Steri-Strips Assess that patient has met discharge criteria.* Discontinue saline lock.
IVs	IV fluids D₅ ½ NSS+ MVI	IV convert to saline lock	Continue saline lock	D
Medication	PCA (0.5 mg basal rate)	Discontinue PCA. PO analgesia Resume routine home meds.	PO analgesia Preoperative meds	PO analgesia Preoperative meds
Diet/GI	Discontinue NG tube per guidelines: (Clamp tube at 8 a.m. if no N/V and residual less than 200 mL, D/C tube at 1200.)* (Check with doctor first.)	Clear liquids if+bm/flatus. Advance to postoperative diet if tolerating clears (at least one tray of clear liquids).	House	House
Activity	Ambulate four times/day with abdominal binder.* May shower Physical therapy b.i.d.	Ambulate at least four times/day with abdominal binder.* May shower Physical therapy b.i.d.	Ambulate at least four times/day with abdominal binder.* May shower Physical therapy b.i.d.	
Teaching	Reinforce preoperative teaching.* Patient and family education p.r.n.* Re: family screening	Reinforce preoperative teaching.* Patient and family education p.r.n.* Re: family screening Begin discharge teaching.	Reinforce preoperative teaching.* Patient and family education p.r.n.* Discharge teaching re: reportable s/s, follow-up, and wound care*	Review all discharge instructions and Rx including* follow-up appointments with surgeon within 3 weeks with oncologist within 1 month if indicated.

The pathway lists key events that must occur before the patient's discharge date.

| **KEY:** * = NSG Activities V = Variance N = No Var. | 1. 2. 3. V V V Ⓝ Ⓝ Ⓝ | 1. 2. 3. V V V Ⓝ Ⓝ Ⓝ | 1. 2. 3. V V V Ⓝ Ⓝ Ⓝ | 1. 2. 3. V V V Ⓝ Ⓝ N |
| **Signatures:** | 1. *A. McCarthy, RN* 2. *R. Mayer, Rn* 3. *L. Waters, RN* | 1. *A. McCarthy, RN* 2. *R. Mayer, Rn* 3. *L. Waters, RN* | 1. *L. Singer, RN* 2. *J. Smith, RN* 3. *P. Joseph, RN* | 1. *L. Singer, RN* 2. *J. Smith, RN* 3. |

Hospice care

Hospice programs also use care plans for their patients. In this setting, the care plan is prepared by an interprofessional team comprising nurses, certified nursing assistants, physicians, therapists, clergy, volunteers, bereavement counselors, and social workers. It's reviewed daily and updated every 2 weeks. (For inpatient hospice patients, care plans may be reviewed on a weekly basis.) All hospice programs, regardless of the setting, must follow Medicare rules and regulations if they want to accept patients under the Medicare hospice benefit program.

Creating care plans: a summary

As previously discussed, everything you do as a nurse focuses on the nursing process, and care plans are a natural extension of that process. Your patient's care plan is a summary of his problems, his goals, and the care he receives. It's also your key to helping him achieve wellness.

Revisiting the nursing process

You'll start developing your care plan beginning with your patient's initial assessment. This is when you'll talk with the patient and his family members to gather subjective and objective data, perform a physical examination, and obtain the medical history.

Taking it step-by-step

From all this information, you'll develop your nursing diagnoses, collaborate with the patient to identify his outcome goals, and begin planning interventions to achieve those goals. The plan you come up with—the nursing care plan—directs your patient care from that moment forward.

EVALUATION
IMPLEMENTATION
PLANNING
NURSING DIAGNOSIS
ASSESSMENT

Why you do what you do

As a student, remember to include a scientific, evidence-based rationale (reason) and cite the reference source, as appropriate, for each intervention. The scientific rationale is the "why" behind the "what."

Why is it necessary to ambulate a surgical patient on the first postoperative day? Why should you assess lung sounds every 4 hours if your patient has heart failure? Right now, you're learning the answers to these and other questions in your classroom setting and by researching journals and other textbooks. With each new patient, you'll acquire more and more knowledge and hone your critical thinking skills. Soon such questions, and their corresponding scientific rationales, will become second nature to you.

As a practicing nurse, you won't include scientific rationales in the patient's care plan. But don't think this lets you off the hook! Nursing is continually evolving, just like health care delivery in general. Long-trusted techniques and standards of care may be rejected as research shows better ways to accomplish the same tasks. Throughout your career, you'll need to stay up-to-date with the latest evidence-based practice and standards of care. In fact, many states require registered nurses to have several continuing education credits to renew their nursing licenses.

Evaluating and reassessing at every turn

Keep in mind that, as you perform each intervention, you'll need to evaluate your patient's condition and response to the intervention. In some cases, these responses will require you to change the care plan accordingly. For example, your patient may not be able to walk the distance specified in his care plan or his pneumonia may be clearing up and you won't need to assess his breath sounds as frequently as specified in the care plan. Such changes mean re-examining the interventions and expected outcomes and making necessary modifications if the patient hasn't yet achieved his outcome goal.

Sample care plans and concept maps

During your rotations, you'll probably care for patients in maternity, pediatric, psychiatric, and medical-surgical settings. On the pages that follow, you'll find sample patient scenarios, with corresponding concept maps and care plans, for some of these settings. These care plans and concept maps are included to help you analyze how a care plan comes together. As you review these sample plans, try to think of other possible diagnoses, outcomes, and interventions that might be appropriate for these patients.

Welcome, baby!

An 18-year-old female, Patricia Thomas, just gave birth to an 8-lb, 2-oz baby boy via cesarean delivery. She isn't married, but her boyfriend is present. Her parents are also present but are visibly tense. The patient's vital signs are stable, but she's in pain. She states that she wants to breast-feed the baby, so you assist her in turning on her side and you position the baby beside her. You show her how to get the baby to latch on, but the young mother is having difficulty and becomes frustrated. "Don't give up," says the boyfriend.

This patient's care plan focuses on the nursing diagnoses *Deficient knowledge (breast-feeding)* and *Acute pain*. The concept map for this patient might look like this:

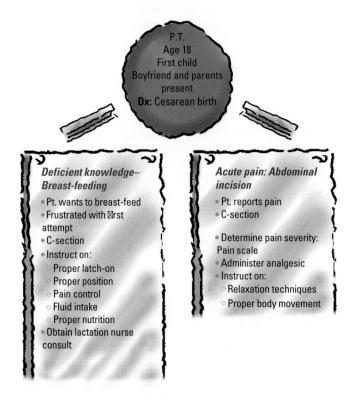

See *Sample maternal-neonatal care plan* to see what the care plan might look like.

Sample maternal-neonatal care plan

Here's an example of what the care plan might look like for the maternal patient described in the text.

Nursing diagnosis 1

Deficient knowledge (breast-feeding) related to unfamiliarity as evidenced by being a first-time mother who's new to breast-feeding

Outcome

The mother will demonstrate proper latching-on technique and nursing positions before discharge. The baby will have a good suck reflex and audible swallowing.

Interventions	Rationale
1. Teach the mother proper latch-on technique.	1. Proper latch-on ensures proper sucking by infant, which in turn affects milk supply.
2. Instruct the mother on the different nursing positions, especially the sidelying and football hold positions, which are best for post-cesarean delivery patients.	2. Positioning to decrease strain on the incision and increase neonatal comfort and safety is conducive to letdown.
3. Offer and administer pain medications as needed.	3. Being pain free helps the mother relax and promotes the letdown reflex.
4. Encourage the mother to drink at least eight glasses of fluid per day.	4. Good hydration is essential for a healthy milk supply.
5. Encourage the mother to increase her caloric intake.	5. Breast-feeding mothers need to consume 500 calories more per day than they did when they were pregnant to help with milk production.
6. Obtain an order for a lactation nurse if needed.	6. Lactation nurses specialize in dealing with breast-feeding problems and offering correct information.

Nursing diagnosis 2

Post-operative pain due to caesarian section as evidenced by patient report and nonverbal behavior

Outcome

The mother will verbalize decreased pain each day and minimal pain by discharge.

Interventions	Rationale
1. Assess and document severity of pain every shift and as needed, using a 0 to 10 pain scale.	1. Knowing the patient's pain severity assists in providing the correct type and dose of pain medication.
2. Administer pain medication as ordered.	2. Pain medications help alleviate pain and promote rest.
3. Teach the mother not to wait for pain to get severe before asking for pain medication.	3. Severe pain may require more medication or more time to become alleviated.
4. Teach the mother relaxation techniques.	4. Relaxation techniques help lessen pain perception and can assist with coping with stress at home.
5. Teach the mother the proper techniques for getting out of a chair and bed.	5. Proper movements help minimize discomfort and pain when getting up.

Feeling the blues

A 65-year-old female, Julie Blue, is admitted with depression and inadequate nutrition due to lack of eating. Her husband of 45 years passed away unexpectedly 1 year ago, and she hasn't been coping well with his death. Her daughter brought her to the hospital because she couldn't get her mother to eat, bathe, get out of bed, or brush her hair for 2 weeks.

The patient states, "I just can't go on without my husband. He did everything." The daughter also tells the nurse that the electric and water have been turned off because her mother keeps forgetting to pay the bills.

The concept map for this patient might look like this:

J.B.
Age 65
Widowed 1 year,
married 45 years
Daughter present
Dx: Major depression;
inadequate nutrition

Ineffective coping
• Decreased self-care
• Decreased appetite
• S&S depressed mood
• Pt. states: "I can't cope"
• Not handling ⊠nances

• Encourage verbalization of feelings
• Use active listening
• Administer antidepressants as ordered
• Promote independence
• Teach problem-solving tools
• Consult pastoral care and social services

Complicated grieving
• Spouse died 1 year ago
• Deteriorating mood and self-care since loss

• Examine factors prolonging grief
• Encourage verbalization of feelings
• Identify support systems
• Set realistic goals

See *Sample psychiatric care plan,* page 173, to see what the care plan might look like.

Boy, oh boy!

A 10-year-old boy with cystic fibrosis, Bobby Young, is admitted to the hospital with an upper respiratory tract infection and fever. His oral temperature is 101.6°F. He's coughing up copious amounts of

Sample psychiatric care plan

Here's an example of what the care plan might look like for the patient described in the text.

Nursing diagnosis 1

Ineffective coping related to sudden death of spouse 1 year ago as evidenced by lack of self-care and verbalization of inability to cope

Outcome

The patient will verbalize feelings about the death of her husband and demonstrate new coping mechanisms by discharge.

Interventions	Rationale
1. Encourage the patient to talk about her feelings.	1. Verbalizing feelings makes the patient and others aware of what the patient is going through.
2. Use active listening and a calm, unhurried manner.	2. This approach conveys to the patient your concern and willingness to listen.
3. Administer antidepressants as ordered.	3. Medications may be essential to assist the patient with the mood disorder.
4. Encourage the patient to independently perform at least one activity of daily living each day.	4. Self-care helps improve patient outlook, self-worth, and independence.
5. Teach the patient problem-solving tools, such as the step-by-step approach and weighing advantages and disadvantages.	5. Knowledge of problem-solving tools assists with day-to-day activities on discharge.
6. Allow the patient time to solve at least one simple problem per day on her own (such as what to eat or wear).	6. Successful problem solving promotes independence and self-confidence.
7. Assist the patient in identifying problems or issues that she can't control or change.	7. Helping the patient realize her limitations decreases stress and feelings of incompetence.
8. Obtain an order for consults with pastoral care and social services, as needed.	8. Spiritual guidance or assistance with other issues may be helpful as the patient identifies issues of concern.

Nursing diagnosis 2

Complicated grieving related to loss of spouse as evidenced by depression, social isolation, inability to cope with ADLs

Outcome

The patient will verbalize feelings of grief and demonstrate use of new coping methods for managing her feelings by discharge.

Interventions	Rationale
1. Assess for factors that are prolonging the grieving process.	1. Identifying a problem will help to solve it.
2. Encourage the patient to talk about feelings of grief, anger, and depression in individual and group therapy sessions.	2. Acknowledging feelings is first step to finding ways to deal with them.
3. Assist the patient in identifying her support systems.	3. Support systems can help patient in time of emotional need.
4. Discuss with the patient methods to cope with stresses such as focusing on living life "one day at a time."	4. Planning too far ahead can increase stress as new coping skills are developed.
5. Assist the patient in setting realistic goals.	5. Accomplishing short-term goals will help her gain a sense of control of her life.

yellowish green sputum. He's talkative but tires easily. His mother says his symptoms started about 2 days ago; she noticed that he'd gone to bed earlier because he was tired and that he appeared to be coughing more in the evening. She gave him an extra breathing treatment last night, but it didn't seem to help. The patient has been drinking his fluids well and taking his medications without any problems. His lung sounds on admission reveal rhonchi throughout the lower lobes. He has no acute shortness of breath and no other problems. His chest X-ray reveals no significant findings. The concept map for this patient might look like this:

B.Y.
Age 10
Mother present
Cystic fibrosis
DX: Upper respiratory tract infection

Ineffective airway clearance
- Increased fatigue
- Fever 101.6°F
- Increased sputum production
- Sputum color change to yellowish green
- Assess lung sounds
- Monitor sputum
- Check VS
- Give antibiotics
- Teach cleaning of respiratory equipment
- Advise flu shot
- Instruct to avoid crowds

Ineffective protection
- Chronic multisystem disorder with lung involvement
- Teach hand washing
- Instruct to avoid crowds
- Maintain good health habits

See *Sample pediatric care plan* to see what the care plan might look like. Note that this care plan addresses the patient's present infection and ongoing infection risk.

And many more...

Throughout your nursing career, you're likely to create or encounter plenty of nursing care plans. Using the previous examples, and everything you've learned about care planning in this book, see if you can create your own care plan for the medical-surgical patient described in the *On the case* quiz on page 176.

Sample pediatric care plan

Here's an example of what the care plan might look like for the patient described in the text.

Nursing diagnosis 1
Ineffective airway clearance related to acute respiratory infection as evidenced by increased amount of sputum, yellowish-green sputum color, increased fatigue, and fever

Outcome
The patient will demonstrate clear lung sounds, lack of fever, and return to baseline energy level by discharge.

Interventions	Rationale
1. Assess lung sounds and respiratory pattern at beginning of every shift and as needed.	1. Early recognition of worsening condition leads to early treatment and improved patient outcomes.
2. Assess amount, color, and consistency of sputum every shift.	2. Increased amounts, thickening, and continued color change of sputum can indicate worsening infection.
3. Assess vital signs every shift. Report deteriorating findings to the practitioner.	3. Increasing temperature and respirations indicate poor response to treatment.
4. Position the patient in a position of comfort with the head of bed in a semi-Fowler's position	4. Assuming a position of comfort such as semi-Fowler's position promotes rest and breathing for the client.
5. Place a high-humidity face mask with or without oxygen as ordered.	5. Humidification of oxygen delivers high humidity to the tracheobronchial tree, helps liquefy secretions, and relieves tracheobronchial irritation.
6. Help the patient perform deep breathing and controlled coughing techniques.	6. Coughing and deep breathing mobilizes pulmonary secretions so that the patient can expectorate sputum.
7. Provide 2,000 mL of fluids every day. Ask the patient about fluid preferences.	7. Increasing hydration will thin and loosen pulmonary secretions.
8. Encourage activity and ambulation as tolerated by the patient.	8. Mobilizing the patient will promote expectoration of secretions.
9. Administer antibiotics as ordered.	9. Antibiotics help to fight infection.
10. Administer anti-inflammatory medications as ordered.	10. Anti-inflammatory medications may be prescribed for the patient. Corticosteroids may be used to treat an acute inflammation. Nonsteroidal anti-inflammatory agents may be prescribed on a routine basis to slow loss of lung function.
11. Teach the patient and family proper cleaning of respiratory equipment.	11. Proper cleaning of respiratory equipment helps to prevent bacterial growth.
12. Teach the patient the importance of avoiding crowds during flu season and getting flu vaccine yearly.	12. Cystic fibrosis puts the patient at higher risk for infection. Avoiding crowds limits exposure to the flu. Yearly flu vaccine provides additional protection.
13. Collaborate with respiratory therapy regarding postural drainage, percussion, and vibration as ordered.	13. Chest physiotherapy will loosen and mobilize secretions.

(continued)

Sample pediatric care plan (*continued*)

Nursing diagnosis 2

Ineffective protection related to chronic medical condition characterized by respiratory infections as evidenced by ongoing sputum production, enzymatic disorder, and increased risk of infection

Outcome

The patient and family will verbalize understanding of instructions on risk reduction by discharge.

Interventions	Rationale
1. Reinforce with the patient and family that proactive handwashing is a major defense against secondary infection.	1. Handwashing prevents incidental exposure to infection.
2. Teach the patient and family to actively avoid crowded environments during flu season and to avoid people who are ill.	2. Active attention to environmental risks can decrease exposure to infectious agents.
3. Teach the patient to maintain healthy rest, nutrition, and lung maintenance programs.	3. Healthy daily habits promote increased resistance to infectious agents.

On the case

Case study background

A 56-year-old male is admitted to the medical-surgical unit with chronic obstructive pulmonary disease (COPD) and pneumonia. He has shortness of breath and audible wheezes and appears anxious. He's unable to answer all of the medical history questions, so his wife answers for him while he sits, leaning over the bedside table. She says he has been coughing up more sputum the past 3 days and that it's green in color. His vital signs are oral temperature 99.2°F, pulse 115 beats/minute, respirations 28 breaths/minute and labored with accessory muscle use, and blood pressure 142/68 mm Hg. During the physical examination, the nurse notes 2+ edema of both feet and an irregular heartbeat.

His arterial blood gas results in the emergency department (ED) were pH 7.30, $PaCO_2$ 65 mm Hg, PaO_2 55 mm Hg, HCO_3^- 30 mEq/L, and SaO_2 88%. The ED placed the patient on 24% oxygen by VentiMask, IV D_5W at 50 mL/hour, methylprednisolone sodium succinate (Solu-Medrol) 40 mg IV q6h, erythromycin 500 mg IV q6h, breathing treatments q4h, bed rest, and nothing-by-mouth status.

Critical thinking exercise

1. Complete a three-diagnosis care plan, including at least three interventions and rationales for each diagnosis, for this medical-surgical patient.

Nursing diagnosis 1

Outcome

_____

Interventions	Rationale
1. _____	1. _____
2. _____	2. _____
3. _____	3. _____

Nursing diagnosis 2

Outcome

_____

Interventions	Rationale
1. _____	1. _____
2. _____	2. _____
3. _____	3. _____

Nursing diagnosis 3

Outcome

_____

Interventions	Rationale
1. _____	1. _____
2. _____	2. _____
3. _____	3. _____

Answer key

1. Five potential nursing diagnoses for this patient are given in the care plan on pages 178 to 181. See how many of your diagnoses, outcomes, and interventions match. Did you think of a different diagnosis? You could be right! As long as your care plan was consistent with what you know about COPD and pneumonia, met the patient's profile, and was logically thought out, you've probably developed a good care plan.

Nursing diagnosis 1

Impaired gas exchange related to inadequate ventilation and excessive mucus production as evidenced by wheezes and labored respirations with accessory muscle use

Outcome

The patient will maintain adequate gas exchange as evidenced by return of arterial blood gas (ABG) values back to his baseline by discharge.

Interventions	Rationale
1. Assess and document respiratory rate and pattern, pulse oximetry every shift, and ABGs as ordered. Report changes.	1. Early recognition of deteriorating respiratory function can improve patient outcomes.
2. Auscultate breath sounds every 2 hours on even hours.	2. If crackles and wheezes are present, then the patient may experience hypoxia or increasing hypoxia.
3. Monitor the patient's behavior and mental status on even hours.	3. Patient may exhibit restlessness, agitation, confusion and/or lethargy when hypoxic.
4. Maintain low-flow oxygen therapy as ordered.	4. Oxygen therapy helps to correct hypoxemia. High oxygen saturation levels may diminish a COPD patient's respiratory drive and cause further retention of carbon dioxide.
5. Administer bronchodilators as ordered. Watch for adverse effects of tachycardia and arrhythmias.	5. Bronchodilators relax bronchial smooth muscle, improving air flow.
6. Assist the patient to high Fowler's position as needed.	6. High Fowler's position promotes fuller lung expansion.
7. Encourage the patient to take deep breaths and cough.	7. Taking deep breaths and coughing will promote lung expansion.
8. Teach the patient pursed lip breathing.	8. Pursed lip breathing slows the patient's expiration, helps to prevent collapse of the small airways, and control the rate of respirations. It also promotes relaxation, particularly when the patient may be dyspneic.

Nursing diagnosis 2
Ineffective airway clearance related to increased sputum production as evidenced by increased sputum, wheezes, and patient report of shortness of breath

Outcome
The patient will have a patent airway as evidenced by decreased amounts of mucus by discharge.

Interventions	Rationale
1. Assess lung sounds and respiratory rate and pattern every 4 hours and as needed.	**1.** Rhonchi decrease the airflow patency of large airways. Increased respiratory rate and labored breathing are signs of respiratory distress due to mucus plug or inadequate airway clearance.
2. Assess amount, color, and consistency of sputum every shift.	**2.** Increased amounts, thickening, and continued color change of sputum can indicate worsening infection.
3. Assess vital signs every shift and report deteriorating findings to the practitioner.	**3.** Increasing temperature, heart rate, and respirations indicates poor response to treatment.
4. Place the patient in a position of comfort, such as semi-Fowler's position.	**4.** Assuming a position of comfort such as semi-Fowler's position promotes rest and breathing for the client.
5. Administer antibiotics as ordered.	**5.** Antibiotics help to fight infection.
6. Administer bronchodilators and steroids as ordered.	**6.** Relaxation of the tracheobronchial tree will aid in the mobilization of secretions.
7. Teach the patient effective coughing techniques.	**7.** Proper coughing techniques loosen mucus and ease expectoration, helping to conserve patient energy.
8. Teach the patient about adequate hydration (drinking at least six 8-oz glasses of fluid per day, unless contraindicated).	**8.** Adequate hydration helps to thin secretions.
9. Perform chest physiotherapy, if ordered.	**9.** Chest physiotherapy helps to loosen secretions.
10. Monitor the patient's performance of incentive spirometry as ordered.	**10.** Incentive spirometry helps promote lung expansion.
11. Suction the patient to remove mucus from the back of the throat and mouth.	**11.** Thick secretions are difficult to cough out and the patient may not have the energy to do so.

Nursing diagnosis 3
Activity intolerance related to dyspnea and inadequate oxygenation as evidenced by labored respirations with accessory muscle use and patient report of shortness of breath

Outcome
The patient will perform activities of daily living (ADLs) with minimal assistance by discharge.

Interventions	Rationale
1. Monitor the severity of dyspnea and oxygen saturation during patient activity.	**1.** Activity increases oxygen demand. Assessing these variables reveals the patient's tolerance of ADLs.

(*continued*)

Interventions	Rationale
2. Maintain oxygen therapy with activity as needed.	2. Activity increases oxygen demand of the muscles. Oxygen therapy helps alleviate hypoxemia and helps to improve activity tolerance.
3. Schedule activities after breathing treatments.	3. Breathing treatments maximize lung function and improve activity tolerance.
4. Help the patient to gradually increase activities every day.	4. A gradual, steady increase in activity helps to improve respiratory and cardiac condition.
5. Teach the patient to stop or change any activity that causes worsening dyspnea with increased heart rate.	5. Worsening dyspnea with increased heart rate signals activity intolerance, which increases the patient's oxygen demand.
6. Teach the patient to avoid factors that increase oxygen demand, such as smoking, temperature extremes, excess weight, and stress.	6. An increase in oxygen demand increases cardiac workload
7. Teach the patient energy conservation techniques.	7. Using less energy to accomplish tasks will decrease oxygen demand.
8. Teach the patient pursed lip and diaphragmatic breathing techniques and explain that he should use these techniques during activities.	8. These techniques allow the patient to accomplish more with the limited energy he has and maximize lung function.

Nursing diagnosis 4
Risk for infection related to ineffective clearance of secretions

Outcome
The patient will verbalize methods to reduce risk of infection by discharge.

Interventions	Rationale
1. Teach the patient proper hand-washing technique.	1. Good handwashing is the single most important defense against the spread of infection.
2. Teach the patient how to care for and clean respiratory equipment at home.	2. Standing water in respiratory equipment can be a source of bacterial growth.
3. Teach the patient and family early signs of infection (increased sputum, change in sputum color, and increased dyspnea).	3. Early detection leads to early treatment and decreases the risk of complications.
4. Teach the patient to maintain healthy rest, nutrition, and lung maintenance programs.	4. Healthy daily habits promote increased resistance to infectious agents.
5. Teach the patient about the importance of getting a yearly flu vaccine.	5. The flu vaccine provides some immunity from infection.

Nursing diagnosis 5
Anxiety related to dyspnea as evidenced by rapid and labored respirations and patient report of shortness of breath

Outcome
The patient will verbalize decreased feelings of anxiety within 48 hours of admission.

Interventions	Rationale
1. Assess the patient's level of anxiety and physical reactions to the anxiety.	1. When patients who have shortness of breath experience anxiety, the patients may experience increased shortness of breath.
2. Stay with the patient during episodes of shortness of breath and provide reassurance.	2. Having someone present during these episodes decreases patient anxiety.
3. Encourage the use of breathing techniques during episodes of shortness of breath and anxiety.	3. Successful use of breathing techniques helps to reduce anxiety.
4. Maintain a calm environment.	4. A calm environment promotes relaxation.
5. Teach the patient relaxation techniques, such as guided imagery and visualization.	5. Relaxation techniques help to reduce anxiety.

Selected references

Alfaro-LeFevre, R. (2014). *Applying nursing process*. Philadelphia, PA: Wolters Kluwer.

American Nurse Association. (2015). *Nursing scope and standards of performance and standards of clinical practice* (3rd ed.). Silver Spring, MD: nursesbooks.org.

Hinkle, J., & Cheever, K. (2014). *Brunner & Suddarth's textbook of medical-surgical nursing* (13th ed.). New York: Lippincott Williams & Wilkins.

Nettina, S. (2014). *Lippincott's manual of nursing practice* (10th ed.). New York: Lippincott Williams & Wilkins.

2017 National Patient Safety Goals: https://www.jointcommission.org/standards_information/npsgs.aspx

Taylor, C., & Lillis, P. (2014). *Fundamentals of nursing; the art and science of person-centered nursing care* (8th ed.). Philadelphia, PA: Lippincott Williams & Wilkins.

Part II

Nursing diagnoses by medical diagnosis

Chapter 8

Medical-surgical diagnoses

Just the facts

In this chapter, you'll learn:

◆ nursing diagnoses that correlate with common medical-surgical medical diagnoses.

A look at medical-surgical diagnoses

This chapter covers medical-surgical problems that are common in adult patients. Each entry provides a list of a few of the major nursing diagnoses and related factors to be considered after your assessment of a patient with the particular medical diagnosis. Remember that the nursing diagnoses listed here represent the needs most commonly associated with the medical condition; your patient may have different needs.

Remember that your nursing diagnoses should be specific to the patient—not necessarily the disorder.

Abdominal aortic aneurysm repair

- Acute pain related to surgical tissue trauma
- Anxiety related to threat to health status
- Decreased cardiac output related to:
  - changes in intravascular volume
  - increased systemic vascular resistance
  - third-space fluid shift
- Deficient knowledge (preoperative and postoperative care) related to newly identified need for aortic surgery
- Impaired skin integrity related to surgical incision
- Ineffective breathing pattern related to:
  - effects of general anesthesia
  - endotracheal intubation
  - presence of an abdominal incision
- change in activity level and presence of pain

Abdominal injury

- Acute pain related to tissue trauma
- Deficient fluid volume related to active blood loss
- Fear related to unknown diagnosis and prognosis
- Ineffective breathing pattern related to surgical incision
- Risk for adverse reaction to iodinated contrast media related to diagnostic procedure
- Risk for infection related to:
  ○ penetrating wound
  ○ potential bowel rupture

Abdominal injuries may be associated with pain or infection. Look for signs of these related problems in your patient.

Acquired immunodeficiency syndrome

- Deficient fluid volume related to persistent diarrhea associated with opportunistic infections
- Deficient knowledge (symptoms of disease progression, risk factors, transmission of disease, home care, and treatment options) related to lack of exposure to information
- Grieving related to uncertain prognosis and change in health status
- Imbalanced nutrition: Less than body requirements related to:
  ○ anorexia
  ○ diarrhea
  ○ medication adverse effects
  ○ nausea and vomiting
  ○ malabsorption or lack of food intake
- Impaired gas exchange related to:
  ○ respiratory failure
  ○ ventilation-perfusion imbalance
- Impaired oral mucous membrane related to:
  ○ masses
  ○ opportunistic infections
- Impaired physical mobility related to:
  ○ fatigue and weakness
  ○ hypoxemia
  ○ medication adverse effects
- Ineffective airway clearance related to pneumonia
- Ineffective breathing pattern related to fatigue
- Ineffective therapeutic regimen management related to complexity of therapeutic regimen
- Risk for compromised human dignity related to:
  ○ body image
  ○ social isolation
  ○ societal prejudice and stigma
- Risk for impaired skin integrity related to:
  ○ effects of immobility
  ○ medication reactions

- ○ opportunistic disease effects
- ○ poor nutritional status
- Risk for infection related to immunosuppression
- Sexual dysfunction related to:
  - ○ depression
  - ○ fatigue
  - ○ fear of disease transmission
  - ○ fear of rejection
- Social isolation related to:
  - ○ associated societal stigma
  - ○ contacts' fear of being infected
  - ○ depression
  - ○ fear of infection from social contacts

Acute alcohol withdrawal
- Acute confusion related to chemical imbalances
- Imbalanced nutrition: Less than body requirements related to lack of food intake
- Risk for injury related to abrupt withdrawal of alcohol and withdrawal-inducing hallucinations or seizures

Acute poststreptococcal glomerulonephritis
- Activity intolerance related to inadequate tissue oxygenation and inadequate nutritional status
- Acute pain related to inflammatory process
- Decreased cardiac output related to decreased preload
- Excess fluid volume related to altered renal function
- Imbalanced nutrition: Less than body requirements related to proteinuria
- Impaired gas exchange related to decreased lung expansion
- Impaired physical mobility related to altered hemodynamic status
- Risk for constipation related to decreased intake of foods high in fiber and decreased gastrointestinal motility
- Risk for electrolyte imbalance related to inability to excrete fluids
- Risk for infection related to altered immune state
- Risk for injury related to alteration in hemodynamic status

Acute respiratory distress syndrome
- Deficient fluid volume related to active fluid volume loss
- Imbalanced nutrition: Less than body requirements related to inability to ingest food due to mechanical ventilation
- Impaired gas exchange related to alveolocapillary membrane changes
- Impaired skin integrity related to immobility and decreased nutritional intake

- Impaired spontaneous ventilation related to respiratory muscle fatigue
- Impaired verbal communication related to physical barriers of mechanical ventilation
- Ineffective airway clearance related to retained secretions

Acute respiratory failure

- Activity intolerance related to respiratory distress and fatigue
- Anxiety related to sensation of severe shortness of breath
- Bathing, dressing, toileting self-care deficits related to:
  - fatigue with exertion
  - shortness of breath at rest and decreased oxygenation with position changes
- Imbalanced nutrition: Less than body requirements related to shortness of breath
- Impaired gas exchange related to ventilation-perfusion imbalance
- Risk for decreased cardiac tissue perfusion related to impaired transport of oxygen across alveolocapillary membranes
- Risk for suffocation related to respiratory collapse

Acute respiratory distress syndrome can affect everything from gas exchange and fluid volume to skin integrity and verbal communication.

Adrenal hypofunction

- Decreased cardiac output related to altered heart rate
- Deficient fluid volume related to nausea, vomiting, and diarrhea
- Fatigue related to muscle weakness, change in weight, and the stress of the disease process
- Activity intolerance related to hypotension
- Risk for injury related to decreased ability to mount a sufficient response to stress

Alzheimer's disease

- Bathing, dressing, feeding, toileting self-care deficits related to cognitive impairment
- Caregiver role strain related to the complexity and amount of caregiving tasks
- Chronic confusion related to degenerative loss of cerebral tissue
- Constipation related to:
  - inadequate diet
  - inadequate fluid intake
  - memory loss about toileting behavior
- Imbalanced nutrition: Less than body requirements related to:
  - difficulty swallowing
  - inadequate food intake
  - memory loss
- Impaired memory related to degenerative loss of cerebral tissue
- Impaired verbal communication related to advanced confusion
- Risk for aspiration related to advanced confusion

- Risk for injury related to:
  - agnosia
  - apraxia
  - aphasia
  - wandering behavior
  - confusion and agitation
- Wandering related to cognitive impairment

I can't remember, did you already read the nursing diagnoses that are associated with Alzheimer's disease?

Amputation

- Acute pain related to postoperative tissue, nerve, and bone trauma
- Disturbed body image related to loss of a body part
- Impaired physical mobility related to loss of a body part
- Impaired skin integrity related to traumatic or surgical tissue removal
- Risk for injury related to altered mobility
- Grieving related to amputation and potential for disability

Amblyopia

- Anxiety related to sudden onset of impaired vision
- Compromised family coping related to increased health care needs
- Fear related to sudden onset of impaired vision
- Risk for infection related to alteration in eye integrity
- Risk for injury related to sudden alteration in vision

Amyotrophic lateral sclerosis

- Bowel incontinence related to neuromuscular impairment
- Caregiver role strain related to complexity of care needs
- Death anxiety related to disease prognosis
- Decisional conflict related to decision concerning intubation
- Grieving related to disease prognosis
- Hopelessness related to disease prognosis
- Impaired physical mobility related to muscle atrophy
- Impaired spontaneous ventilation related to respiratory muscle enervation
- Impaired swallowing related to neuromuscular impairment
- Impaired verbal communication related to neuromuscular impairment
- Ineffective airway clearance related to retained secretions
- Ineffective breathing pattern related to neuromuscular impairment
- Ineffective health maintenance related to lack of gross and fine motor skills
- Powerlessness related to disease progression
- Risk for aspiration related to neuromuscular impairment
- Risk for suicide related to terminal illness
- Risk for thermal injury related to neuromuscular impairment

Anaphylaxis

- Death anxiety related to acute respiratory distress
- Decreased cardiac output related to altered heart rate and hypotension
- Impaired gas exchange related to edema of upper respiratory tract
- Risk for ineffective cerebral tissue perfusion related to impaired transport of oxygen across alveolocapillary membranes

Anemia

Fatigue related to low hemoglobin level leaves me feeling exhausted!

- Activity intolerance related to weakness, fatigue, and shortness of breath
- Fatigue related to low hemoglobin level
- Hopelessness related to chronic fatigue and activity intolerance
- Imbalanced nutrition: Less than body requirements related to:
  - anorexia
  - fatigue
  - lack of knowledge of need for specific nutrients (folate, iron, vitamin B_{12})
- Ineffective protection related to decreased oxygen-carrying capacity of blood
- Risk for impaired skin integrity related to:
  - decreased mobility and bed rest
  - tissue hypoxia

Aneurysm, cerebral

- Acute pain related to aneurysm
- Compromised family coping related to unknown prognosis
- Decreased intracranial adaptive capacity related to increased intracranial pressure from brain hemorrhage
- Risk for acute confusion related to moderate bleeding of cerebral artery into the brain

Aneurysm, femoral and popliteal

- Acute pain related to:
  - compression of nerves
  - edema
  - ischemia
- Deficient knowledge (preoperative and postoperative care) related to lack of exposure to information
- Ineffective peripheral tissue perfusion related to thrombus formation and ischemia

Aneurysm, thoracic aortic

- Acute pain related to thoracic aortic aneurysm
- Risk for decreased cardiac tissue perfusion related to aortic insufficiency
- Risk for deficient fluid volume related to compromised regulatory mechanisms

Aneurysm, ventricular

- Death anxiety related to risk of life-threatening rupture
- Decreased cardiac output related to arrhythmias
- Risk for ineffective cerebral tissue perfusion related to heart failure

Angina pectoris

- Activity intolerance related to development of chest pain on exertion
- Anxiety related to situational crisis and shortness of breath and fear of death
- Decreased cardiac output related to reduced stroke volume
- Deficient knowledge (cardiac diagnostic procedures) related to new onset of angina and underlying cardiovascular disease
- Readiness for enhanced management of therapeutic regimen related to perceived ability to reduce cardiovascular risk factors

Angina pectoris can lead some patients to be intolerant of exercise.

Ankylosing spondylitis

- Activity intolerance related to pain and inflammation of joints
- Chronic pain related to deteriorating bone and cartilage of joints
- Deficient diversional activity related to pain, stiffness, imbalance, and limitation of spinal motion

Aortic insufficiency

- Activity intolerance related to imbalances between oxygen supply and demand
- Anxiety related to lack of understanding of medical diagnosis
- Decreased cardiac output related to increased afterload and preload
- Deficient knowledge related to cardiac disease management
- Excess fluid volume related to decreased excretion of water in response to decreased cardiac output
- Fatigue related to inadequate periods of rest
- Fear related to lack of understanding of medical diagnosis
- Impaired gas exchange related to increased pulmonary interstitial fluid accumulation
- Impaired physical mobility related to altered hemodynamic status
- Ineffective coping related to fear and anxiety of medical diagnosis
- Risk for decreased cardiac tissue perfusion related to decreased cardiac output
- Risk for injury related to weakness

Appendicitis

- Acute pain related to inflammatory process
- Nausea related to peritoneal inflammation
- Risk for infection related to:
  - possible rupture of appendix
  - surgical incision

Arterial occlusive disease

- Acute pain related to arterial occlusion
- Deficient knowledge (disease and treatment options) related to lack of exposure to information
- Ineffective peripheral tissue perfusion related to reduced arterial blood flow

Arteriovenous malformation

- Acute pain related to increased intracerebral pressure
- Anxiety related to lack of understanding of diagnosis, tests, and treatments
- Fear related to lack of understanding of diagnosis, tests, and treatment
- Ineffective coping related to fear, anxiety, and depression
- Risk for deficient fluid volume related to increased fluid loss as a result of compensatory mechanism to control intracerebral pressure
- Risk for ineffective cerebral tissue perfusion related to decreased cerebral blood flow from intracerebral hemorrhage
- Risk for injury related to motor and/or visual impairment

Atelectasis

- Anxiety related to shortness of breath
- Impaired gas exchange related to alveolocapillary membrane changes
- Ineffective airway clearance related to excessive mucus

Basal cell epithelioma

- Disturbed body image related to cancerous lesion
- Readiness for enhanced knowledge (prevention) related to willingness to learn how to prevent recurrence
- Readiness for enhanced management of therapeutic regimen (skin care and protective measures) related to willingness to follow necessary medical regimen

Bell's palsy

- Disturbed body image related to unilateral facial weakness
- Social isolation related to disturbed body image, speech, and eating difficulties

Benign prostatic hyperplasia

- Impaired urinary elimination related to obstruction by enlarged prostate
- Risk for deficient fluid volume related to postoperative bleeding
- Sexual dysfunction related to postsurgical recovery time, retrograde ejaculation, and anxiety
- Urinary retention related to blockage by enlarged prostate

Bladder cancer

- Deficient knowledge (disease and treatment options) related to lack of exposure to information
- Fear related to unknown prognosis
- Impaired tissue integrity related to radiation or chemotherapy
- Impaired urinary elimination related to bladder irritability and pain
- Risk for adverse reaction to iodinated contrast media related to diagnostic procedure
- Situational low self-esteem (postoperative) related to self-consciousness and disturbed self-image after urinary diversion surgery
- Body image disturbance related to urinary diversion surgery

Blastomycosis

- Acute pain related to tenderness and swelling of bony lesions
- Hyperthermia related to viral infection of upper respiratory tract
- Impaired skin integrity related to macules or papules on exposed body parts
- Ineffective airway clearance related to respiratory fungal infection

Blastomycosis originates as a respiratory infection but can end up affecting the skin and bones.

Blepharitis

- Disturbed body image related to inflammation of margins of eyelids
- Ineffective family therapeutic regimen management related to ability to manage symptoms
- Impaired comfort related to burning and irritation of eyelid
- Impaired skin integrity related to inflammation

Bone tumor

- Acute pain related to pressure from tumor growth
- Anxiety related to change in health status and surgical treatment
- Impaired physical mobility related to tumor growth or postoperative healing response
- Impaired skin integrity related to surgical incision for tumor removal

Botulism

- Death anxiety related to life-threatening disorder
- Deficient fluid volume related to vomiting and diarrhea
- Ineffective breathing pattern related to respiratory muscle failure

Brain abscess

- Acute pain related to edema and necrosis
- Risk for acute confusion related to neurologic impairment
- Risk for ineffective cerebral tissue perfusion related to edema and necrosis
- Risk for injury related to neurologic impairment

Brain tumor

- Anxiety related to:
  - deterioration of physical and mental function
  - risks of treatment options
- Decreased intracranial adaptive capacity related to brain tissue injury
- Impaired verbal communication related to damage to speech center
- Risk for acute confusion related to tissue damage from brain mass
- Risk for ineffective cerebral tissue perfusion related to location of tumor
- Risk for injury related to increased seizure potential and neuromuscular effects of brain tissue damage

Did someone say brain tumor? Now I'm getting anxious!

Breast cancer

- Decisional conflict (treatment choice) related to risks and potential adverse effects of treatment options
- Disturbed body image related to breast surgery, chemotherapy, or radiation treatment
- Fatigue related to effects of disease and treatments
- Impaired skin integrity related to incision following breast surgery
- Ineffective sexuality patterns related to perceived loss of attractiveness after mastectomy
- Stress overload related to family needs while physically and emotionally taxed

Bronchiectasis

- Imbalanced nutrition: Less than body requirements related to inadequate food intake due to illness
- Ineffective breathing pattern related to chronic abnormal dilation of bronchi and destruction of bronchial walls
- Risk for infection related to repeated damage to bronchial walls

Bronchiolitis obliterans with organizing pneumonia

- Activity intolerance related to fatigue and shortness of breath
- Imbalanced nutrition: Less than body requirements related to inadequate food intake due to disturbed taste and anorexia

- Ineffective airway clearance related to excess secretions from infection
- Ineffective breathing pattern related to inflammation of small airways

Buerger's disease

- Deficient knowledge (disease causes and risks, treatment options) related to new diagnosis
- Disturbed body image related to disease
- Ineffective peripheral tissue perfusion related to decreased blood flow to the feet and legs
- Risk-prone health behavior related to smoking addiction

Burns

- Acute pain related to tissue destruction and exposure of nerves in partially destroyed tissue
- Compromised family coping related to prolonged disease or disability
- Contamination related to infective agents at place of injury
- Disturbed body image related to potential scarring and skin grafting
- Imbalanced nutrition: Less than body requirements related to increased metabolic needs of burn healing
- Impaired gas exchange related to airway burns and carbon monoxide inhalation
- Impaired physical mobility related to movement limitations from scar tissue or burn treatments
- Ineffective peripheral tissue perfusion related to:
  - circumferential eschar formation on arms and legs
  - compartment syndrome
  - vascular disruption
- Powerlessness related to illness
- Risk for deficient fluid volume related to active loss through disrupted skin
- Risk for imbalanced body temperature related to infection
- Risk for impaired skin integrity related to nonadherence of graft and impaired donor site healing
- Risk for infection related to:
  - decreased perfusion
  - exposure to contamination
  - impaired immunologic response
  - loss of protective integument
- Risk for injury related to continued exposure to heat or chemicals

Cancer

- Activity intolerance related to weakness from:
  - altered protein metabolism
  - cachexia
  - hypoxia
  - muscle wasting

- Anxiety related to diagnosis, treatment effects, and prognosis
- Chronic pain related to:
  - chemotherapy adverse effects
  - metastasis
  - primary disease
- Imbalanced nutrition: Less than body requirements related to:
  - anorexia
  - changes in taste sensation
  - stomatitis
- Impaired urinary elimination related to hemorrhagic cystitis from chemotherapy
- Ineffective sexuality patterns related to alterations in body image
- Readiness for enhanced hope related to decreased signs of cancer on repeated testing and healthful changes in lifestyle to decrease risk of recurrence
- Risk for adverse reaction to iodinated contrast media related to diagnostic procedure
- Risk for constipation related to opioid use
- Risk for infection related to immunosuppression from chemotherapy and malnutrition
- Risk for peripheral neurovascular dysfunction related to peripheral neuropathies caused by chemotherapy
- Risk for situational low self-esteem related to:
  - hair loss
  - role changes
  - weight loss
- Sleep deprivation related to:
  - alterations in patterns of elimination
  - anxiety and depression
  - fear of dying while sleeping
  - other sequelae of cancer
  - pain

Patients with cancer can experience imbalanced nutrition as a result of anorexia, changes in taste, and stomatitis.

Candidiasis

- Impaired oral mucous membrane related to fungal infection in mouth
- Impaired skin integrity related to fungal infection
- Ineffective thermoregulation related to systemic infection
- Risk for impaired liver function related to fluconazole (Diflucan) or other specific systemic antifungal agents

Cardiac arrhythmias

- Activity intolerance related to shortness of breath or chest pain when dysrhythmic or drug effects
- Anxiety related to change in health status

- Decreased cardiac output related to altered contractility of heart muscle
- Deficient knowledge (disease and treatment options) related to lack of exposure to information
- Fatigue related to arrhythmias
- Fear related to decreased confidence in health status
- Ineffective coping related to inadequate level of control over illness recurrence
- Risk for decreased cardiac tissue perfusion related to impaired cardiac cycle and blood oxygenation

Cardiac surgery

- Acute confusion related to:
  - anesthesia
  - cerebral ischemia or infarction
  - sensory overload from intensive care unit environment
- Deficient fluid volume related to blood loss
- Deficient knowledge (postoperative care) related to complex therapeutic regimen
- Dysfunctional ventilatory weaning response related to respiratory complications postoperatively
- Impaired gas exchange related to:
  - alveolar collapse
  - increased pulmonary shunt
  - increased secretions
  - pain

Cardiac tamponade

- Decreased cardiac output related to altered preload
- Fear related to life-threatening disorder
- Ineffective breathing pattern related to cardiac tamponade

Cardiogenic shock

- Activity intolerance related to:
  - diminished cardiovascular reserve
  - hypoxemia
  - weakness
- Decreased cardiac output related to heart rate abnormalities or diminished contractility
- Excess fluid volume related to compromised regulatory mechanisms
- Impaired gas exchange related to ventilation-perfusion imbalance

Cardiomyopathy

- Activity intolerance related to cardiopulmonary dysfunction
- Acute pain related to decreased tissue perfusion

- Anxiety related to:
  - deterioration in health status
  - lack of understanding of diagnosis and treatment
  - fear of death
- Decreased cardiac output related to:
  - alterations in preload, afterload, heart rate, and contractility
  - arrhythmias and ineffective pump action
- Deficient knowledge (disease and treatment) related to changes in regimen
- Ineffective breathing pattern related to disease process
- Excess fluid volume related to decreased left ventricular compliance
- Fatigue related to inadequate periods of rest
- Impaired gas exchange related to ventilation-perfusion imbalance
- Ineffective coping related to fear and anxiety about disease process
- Risk for ineffective cardiac tissue perfusion related to reduced myocardial contractility

Carotid endarterectomy

- Anxiety related to threat to health status
- Deficient knowledge (procedure) related to unfamiliarity with procedure and hospital protocol
- Impaired gas exchange related to airway obstruction from tracheal compression or aspiration
- Risk for ineffective peripheral tissue perfusion related to decreased blood circulation
- Risk for infection related to surgical incision

Carpal tunnel syndrome

- Acute pain related to nerve compression
- Bathing or hygiene self-care deficit related to pain
- Risk for peripheral neurovascular dysfunction related to disease process

Cataract

- Deficient knowledge (disease and treatment options) related to lack of exposure to information
- Impaired physical mobility related to fear of injury
- Risk for injury related to impaired vision

Cerebral contusion

- Acute pain related to headache after trauma
- Risk for acute confusion related to brain injury
- Risk for adverse reaction to iodinated contrast media related to diagnostic procedure

Disturbances in auditory, olfactory, and visual perception can result from cerebral contusion.

- Risk for ineffective cerebral tissue perfusion related to bruising of brain tissue
- Risk for injury related to brain injury

Cervical cancer

- Acute pain related to tumor invasion
- Deficient knowledge (disease and treatment options) related to lack of exposure to information
- Disturbed body image related to weight loss
- Fatigue related to cancer process and treatment effects
- Sexual dysfunction related to postcoital pain, discharge, and bleeding

Chest injury, blunt

- Acute pain related to injury
- Anxiety related to impaired oxygenation and pain
- Impaired spontaneous ventilation related to blunt trauma
- Ineffective breathing pattern related to chest wall injury

Chlamydia

- Deficient knowledge (disease and treatment options) related to lack of information on sexually transmitted diseases
- Ineffective sexuality patterns related to fear of spreading infection
- Risk for infection related to untreated partners

Cholecystectomy

- Acute pain related to gallbladder inflammation
- Imbalanced nutrition: Less than body requirements related to:
  - altered lipid metabolism
  - increased nutritional needs during healing
  - nasogastric (NG) suction
  - postoperative nothing-by-mouth (NPO) status
  - preoperative nausea and vomiting
- Impaired oral mucous membrane related to NPO status and possible NG suction
- Ineffective breathing pattern related to pain from high abdominal incision
- Risk for infection (postoperative) related to obstruction of external biliary drainage tube

Cholelithiasis, cholecystitis

- Acute pain related to gallbladder inflammation or presence of stones
- Imbalanced nutrition: Less than body requirements related to attacks following meals
- Risk for infection related to complications of disease

Chronic alcoholism

- Dysfunctional family processes: Alcoholism related to alcohol abuse
- Imbalanced nutrition: Less than body requirements related to lack of food intake
- Ineffective coping related to:
  - anger
  - denial
  - dependence
  - chronic illness
  - PTSD
- Ineffective therapeutic regimen management related to denial of problem
- Risk for impaired liver function related to alcohol intake
- Risk for other-directed violence related to:
  - disorientation
  - impaired judgment
- Risk-prone health behavior related to alcohol abuse

Chronic fatigue and immune dysfunction syndrome

- Fatigue related to illness and chronic stress
- Hopelessness related to chronic illness
- Sleep deprivation related to internal factors

Chronic obstructive pulmonary disease

- Activity intolerance related to shortness of breath
- Adult failure to thrive related to fatigue and chronic dyspnea of severe disease
- Deficient knowledge (disease processes and treatment) related to complexity of disorder
- Imbalanced nutrition: Less than body requirements related to shortness of breath during and after meals
- Impaired gas exchange related to impaired excretion of carbon dioxide
- Impaired home maintenance related to inadequate support systems and inability to do tasks due to disease process
- Ineffective breathing pattern related to fatigue or blunting of respiratory drive
- Ineffective sexuality patterns related to:
  - adverse reactions to medications
  - change in body image
  - change in relationship with spouse or partner
  - deconditioning
  - shortness of breath

- Insomnia related to:
  - anxiety
  - bronchodilator's stimulant effect
  - depression
  - shortness of breath

Cirrhosis

- Dysfunctional family processes: Alcoholism related to alcohol addiction
- Excess fluid volume related to fluid retention
- Imbalanced nutrition: Less than body requirements related to:
  - GI symptoms (anorexia, nausea, vomiting, diarrhea)
  - inability to absorb nutrients
- Impaired gas exchange related to ventilation-perfusion imbalance
- Risk for acute confusion related to increasing ammonia levels
- Risk for impaired liver function related to alcohol addiction
- Risk for impaired skin integrity related to edema and pruritus
- Risk for injury related to esophageal variceal hemorrhage
- Knowledge deficit related to cognitive changes of hepatic encephalopathy

Clostridium difficile infection

- Anxiety related to change in health status
- Risk for deficient fluid volume related to diarrhea
- Risk for impaired skin integrity related to diarrhea
- Risk for infection related to inadequate defenses

Cold injury

- Deficient knowledge (prevention of cold injury) related to inexperience with excessive cold
- Hypothermia related to cold injury
- Risk for impaired skin integrity related to frostbite

Colorectal cancer

- Constipation related to GI obstruction
- Diarrhea related to inflammation or malabsorption
- Fatigue related to malnutrition or anemia
- Imbalanced nutrition: Less than body requirements related to inability to absorb nutrients
- Risk for adverse reaction to iodinated contrast media related to diagnostic procedure
- Risk for deficient fluid volume related to diarrhea or bleeding
- Risk for spiritual distress related to potential life-threatening diagnosis

- Anxiety related to life-threatening illness
- Anxiety related to fear of reoccurrence of disease
- Anxiety related to treatment being ineffective

Colostomy

- Deficient knowledge (care of descending or sigmoid colostomy) related to unfamiliarity with altered bowel procedures
- Disturbed body image related to loss of control over fecal elimination
- Risk for impaired skin integrity related to fecal contamination of skin
- Sexual dysfunction related to change in body image

Concussion

- Acute pain related to head trauma
- Altered thought processes related to head trauma
- Nausea related to blow to the head
- Risk for injury related to dizziness, loss of consciousness, and lethargy

A patient with a concussion is at risk for injuries related to dizziness and lethargy. Now that's a blow to the head!

Conjunctivitis

- Risk for impaired skin integrity related to eye discharge and tearing
- Risk for infection related to contagious disease and ability to spread to other eye or other people
- Risk for situational low self-esteem related to hyperemia of eyes

Cor pulmonale

- Activity intolerance related to:
  - exertional dyspnea
  - tissue hypoxia
- Acute pain related to decreased coronary perfusion
- Anxiety related to lack of understanding of diagnosis and treatment
- Decreased cardiac output related to:
  - decreased stroke volume
  - ineffective ventricular pumping
- Excess fluid volume related to cardiopulmonary dysfunction
- Fatigue related to inadequate periods of rest
- Fear related to lack of understanding of prognosis
- Grieving related to poor prognosis
- Impaired gas exchange related to:
  - interstitial pulmonary fluid accumulation
  - pulmonary capillary destruction
- Ineffective airway clearance related to interstitial pulmonary fluid accumulation
- Ineffective breathing pattern related to increased respiratory rate

Corneal abrasion

- Acute pain related to eye injury
- Disturbed sensory perception (visual) related to eye injury
- Risk for injury related to poor visual acuity and photophobia

Corneal ulcer

- Risk for infection related to inadequate primary defenses
- Risk for injury related to visual blurring

Coronary artery disease

- Anxiety related to angina
- Decreased cardiac output related to diminished coronary blood flow
- Risk for adverse reaction to iodinated contrast media related to diagnostic procedure
- Risk for decreased cardiac tissue perfusion related to atherosclerosis
- Risk for ineffective peripheral tissue perfusion related to decreased blood circulation

Craniotomy

- Deficient knowledge (impending craniotomy) related to lack of exposure to information
- Disturbed body image related to hair loss and possible disruption of motor function
- Risk for deficient fluid volume related to:
  - diuretic therapy
  - fluid restriction
  - GI suction
  - hyperthermia
- Risk for infection related to invasive techniques (surgery, continuous intracranial monitoring, ventricular drains)
- Risk for injury related to:
  - decreased level of consciousness
  - drug therapy
  - effect of anesthetics
  - seizures

Crohn's disease (inflammatory bowel syndrome)

- Acute pain related to bowel inflammation
- Compromised family coping related to chronic disease
- Diarrhea related to bowel inflammation
- Nausea related to bowel inflammation
- Risk for imbalanced fluid volume related to diarrhea
- Risk for infection related to invasive procedures (surgery, home infusions)

- Imbalanced nutrition: Less than body requirements related to lack of food intake due to cramps and pain occurring after meals
- Imbalanced nutrition: Less than body requirements related to malabsorption of nutrients

Cushing's syndrome

- Disturbed body image related to secondary effects of excessive corticosteroid levels
- Excess fluid volume related to high serum corticosteroid levels
- Risk for impaired skin integrity related to secondary effects of medications
- Risk for infection related to the immunosuppressive action of glucocorticoids
- Risk for unstable glucose level related to the anti-insulin properties of glucocorticoids

Defibrillation

- Impaired gas exchange related to cardiopulmonary dysfunction
- Risk for decreased cardiac tissue perfusion related to cardiac arrhythmias
- Risk for impaired skin integrity related to electric current
- Risk for injury related to electric current

Dermabrasion

- Acute pain related to invasive procedure
- Anxiety related to lack of understanding of procedure
- Deficient knowledge related to lack of understanding of procedure
- Fear related to possible outcomes of procedure
- Impaired tissue integrity related to abrading of skin surface
- Risk for infection related to open areas in abraded skin

Dermatitis

- Chronic low self-esteem related to poor body image
- Impaired skin integrity related to inflammation, itching, or lesions of the skin
- Risk for infection related to inadequate primary defenses

Dermatophytosis

- Acute pain related to inflammation
- Impaired skin integrity related to skin infection
- Readiness for enhanced management of therapeutic regimen related to desire to follow through with treatment regimen

Diabetes insipidus

- Constipation related to dehydration
- Deficient fluid volume related to active fluid loss
- Impaired oral mucous membrane related to dehydration

Watch for signs of dehydration in a patient with diabetes insipidus. Fluid volume can be difficult to balance.

Diabetes mellitus

- Compromised family coping related to prolonged disease
- Deficient knowledge (self-care) related to complex chronic disease
- Ineffective therapeutic regimen management related to:
  ○ ineffective coping with chronic disorder
  ○ lack of material resources
  ○ lack of support
- Risk for imbalanced nutrition: More than body requirements related to excessive calorie intake
- Risk for ineffective peripheral tissue perfusion related to decreased blood circulation
- Risk for ineffective renal perfusion related to complications of disease
- Risk for thermal injury related to neuromuscular impairment
- Risk for unstable glucose level related to:
  ○ inadequate endogenous insulin (type 1)
  ○ inadequate endogenous insulin and insulin resistance (type 2)

Diabetic ketoacidosis

- Deficient fluid volume related to osmotic diuresis or vomiting
- Deficient knowledge (self-care) related to lack of exposure to complex disease and therapy information
- Risk for injury related to:
  ○ acidosis
  ○ cerebral dehydration
  ○ decreased perfusion
  ○ hypoxemia
- Risk for unstable glucose level related to decreased cellular glucose uptake and use

Dislocation and subluxation

- Acute pain related to damage to tissue
- Anxiety related to pain and treatment
- Impaired physical mobility related to joint injury and pain

Disseminated intravascular coagulation

- Acute pain related to:
  ○ bleeding into organ or joint capsules
  ○ hematomas
  ○ tissue ischemia
- Deficient fluid volume related to hemorrhage
- Fear related to unfamiliarity with hospital environment
- Impaired gas exchange related to hypoxemia
- Impaired skin integrity related to capillary fragility

Diverticulitis

- Acute pain related to:
  - bowel infection or perforation
  - inflammation
- Constipation related to lack of roughage in diet
- Deficient fluid volume related to active loss and poor intake
- Diarrhea related to inflammation and infection

Drug overdose

- Hopelessness related to:
  - emotional disorganization
  - inadequate resources or support system
  - low self-esteem
- Ineffective airway clearance related to:
  - decreased or absent gag reflex
  - lavage procedures
  - obstruction by tongue
  - reduced alertness
  - vomiting
- Risk-prone health behavior related to drug addiction

Duodenal ulcer

- Chronic pain related to:
  - excessive motility of upper GI tract
  - increased hydrochloric acid secretion
  - increased spasm
  - inflammation of the duodenum
  - intragastric pressure
- Imbalanced nutrition: Less than body requirements related to:
  - dysphagia
  - mouth soreness
  - nausea and vomiting
- Risk for deficient fluid volume related to:
  - diarrhea
  - GI hemorrhage
  - vomiting

Ebola virus infection

- Diarrhea related to viral infection
- Fear related to poor prognosis
- Grieving related to probable death from disease
- Hyperthermia related to infection
- Impaired skin integrity related to diarrhea
- Risk for deficient fluid volume related to diarrhea and hemorrhage

Encephalitis
- Acute pain related to increased intracranial pressure
- Hyperthermia related to infection
- Impaired physical mobility related to possible coma

Endocarditis
- Activity intolerance related to fatigue and weakness
- Decreased cardiac output related to bacterial or fungal invasion of heart
- Hyperthermia related to infection

Endometriosis
- Acute pain related to inflammation and adhesions of endometrial tissue
- Deficient knowledge (disease and treatment options) related to lack of exposure to information
- Sexual dysfunction related to pain and fertility problems

Epididymitis
- Acute pain related to infection
- Risk for infection related to inadequate primary defenses
- Sexual dysfunction related to pain, swelling, and tenderness of groin area

Epilepsy
- Deficient knowledge (disease) related to lack of exposure to information
- Fatigue related to antiseizure medication adverse effect
- Readiness for enhanced management of therapeutic regimen related to desire to follow treatment
- Risk for caregiver role strain related to worry and fear about diagnosis
- Risk for compromised human dignity related to seizures
- Risk for falls related to seizures

Escherichia coli and other Enterobacteriaceae infections
- Acute pain related to crampy diarrhea
- Deficient fluid volume related to loss through diarrhea and vomiting
- Diarrhea related to infection

Esophageal cancer
- Acute pain related to:
  - fistula
  - surgery
  - tumor
  - ulcerative lesions

- Fatigue related to cachexia
- Imbalanced nutrition: Less than body requirements related to dysphagia and pain
- Risk for adverse reaction to iodinated contrast media related to diagnostic procedure
- Risk for aspiration related to dysphagia

Esophageal diverticula

- Imbalanced nutrition: Less than body requirements related to dysphagia and regurgitation
- Impaired swallowing related to dysphagia
- Risk for aspiration related to dysphagia and regurgitation
- Risk for infection related to inadequate primary defenses

Extraocular motor nerve palsy

- Anxiety related to chronic disease
- Bathing/hygiene or feeding self-care deficit related to vision impairment
- Deficient diversional activity related to vision impairment

Fatty liver

- Acute pain related to large, tender liver
- Deficient knowledge (proper diet) related to lack of exposure to information
- Imbalanced nutrition: Less than body requirements related to anorexia and liver inflammation
- Imbalanced nutrition: More than body requirements related to excess fat and calorie consumption
- Risk for impaired liver function related to excess fat accumulation in the liver

Patients with fatty liver are at risk for impaired liver function from too much fat accumulating in the liver. Maybe I should go on a diet…

Femoral popliteal bypass

- Acute pain related to surgical incision
- Impaired physical mobility related to surgery and pre-existing disability
- Impaired skin integrity related to surgical incision and preexisting stasis ulcers
- Ineffective peripheral tissue perfusion related to arterial insufficiency
- Risk for infection related to inadequate primary defenses (broken skin)

Fibromyalgia syndrome

- Activity intolerance related to pain
- Chronic pain related to illness

- Fatigue related to musculoskeletal pain and sleep disturbance
- Insomnia related to pain

Gastric cancer

- Deficient fluid volume related to vomiting and decreased fluid intake
- Delayed surgical recovery related to decreased nutrition, weight loss, possible loss of blood, and compromised immune system
- Imbalanced nutrition: Less than body requirements related to:
  ○ dyspepsia
  ○ epigastric discomfort
  ○ feeling of fullness after eating
- Risk for spiritual distress related to cancer diagnosis and prognosis

Gastritis

- Acute pain related to inflammation
- Deficient knowledge (prevention and treatment) related to lack of exposure to information about smoking, alcohol use, and dietary factors and to medication use
- Nausea related to gastric irritation
- Readiness for enhanced nutrition related to willingness to ingest nonirritating foods

Gastroenteritis

- Acute pain related to intestinal flu
- Nausea related to bacteria, parasites, and virus in intestine
- Risk for deficient fluid volume related to nausea and vomiting
- Risk for imbalanced body temperature related to infection

Gastroesophageal reflux

- Chronic pain related to reflux of gastric and duodenal contents into esophagus
- Deficient knowledge (treatment options) related to lack information about dietary changes
- Risk for adverse reaction to iodinated contrast media related to diagnostic procedure
- Risk for aspiration related to reflux

Gastrointestinal hemorrhage

- Deficient fluid volume related to active bleeding
- Deficient knowledge (potential recurrent bleeding) related to unfamiliarity with disorder
- Fear related to sight of blood, pain, and distressing physical symptoms

- Risk for injury related to:
  - accumulation of toxins
  - electrolyte imbalance
  - inadequate organ perfusion
  - ulcer perforation
  - undetected bleeding

Glaucoma

- Anxiety related to progression of disease
- Deficient knowledge (eye drops administration procedures) related to lack of previous experience
- Risk for injury related to loss of peripheral vision

Glomerulonephritis

- Excess fluid volume related to oliguria
- Imbalanced nutrition: Less than body requirements related to anorexia
- Risk for ineffective renal perfusion related to disease process
- Risk for infection related to inadequate defenses
- Risk for hypertension related to disease

Goiter

- Disturbed body image related to neck distention
- Impaired swallowing related to swelling and distention of neck
- Ineffective breathing pattern related to compression of trachea

Gonorrhea

- Ineffective sexuality patterns related to fear of spreading infection
- Risk for infection related to inadequate primary resources
- Risk for situational low self-esteem related to infection

Gout

- Activity intolerance related to painful joints
- Acute pain related to urate deposits in joints
- Disturbed body image related to joint deformity
- Risk for dry eye related to reduced quantity or quality of tears to moisten eye

Graft rejection syndrome

- Grieving related to loss of graft
- Ineffective tissue perfusion (peripheral, cardiopulmonary, renal) related to stimulation of the complement cascade with resultant thrombosis and tissue infarction
- Powerlessness related to loss of graft

Granulocytopenia, lymphocytopenia

- Deficient knowledge (disease and treatment options) related to lack of exposure to information
- Fatigue related to low white blood cell (WBC) count
- Hyperthermia related to infection
- Risk for infection related to low WBC count

Guillain–Barré syndrome

- Bathing, feeding, toileting self-care deficit related to muscle weakness and paralysis
- Fear related to sudden onset of illness and possible advancing complications
- Impaired spontaneous ventilation related to muscle weakness and paralysis
- Ineffective airway clearance related to neuromuscular dysfunction
- Risk for urge urinary incontinence related to muscle weakness

Hantavirus pulmonary syndrome

- Hyperthermia related to infection
- Impaired gas exchange related to respiratory failure and ventilation-perfusion imbalance
- Ineffective breathing pattern related to pulmonary infiltrates with respiratory compromise

Headache

- Acute pain related to vascular or muscle contraction
- Fatigue related to headache
- Ineffective coping related to recurrence of headaches

Your patient's hearing loss can affect his ability to hear danger signals in the environment, putting him at risk for injury.

Hearing loss

- Readiness for enhanced communication related to ability to learn ways to communicate without adequate hearing
- Risk for injury related to not hearing danger signs in environment
- Social isolation related to disruption of communication and changes in interpersonal relationships

Heart failure

- Decreased cardiac output related to:
  - altered heart rhythm
  - decreased contractility
  - fluid volume overload
  - increased afterload
- Deficient knowledge (treatment regimen) related to lack of exposure to information

- Excess fluid volume related to:
  - decreased myocardial contractility
  - decreased renal perfusion
  - increased sodium and water retention
- Imbalanced nutrition: Less than body requirements related to decreased appetite and unpalatability of low-sodium diet
- Ineffective breathing pattern related to fatigue
- Ineffective therapeutic regimen management related to:
  - complexity of regimen
  - health beliefs
  - negative relationship with caregivers
- Powerlessness related to illness

Heart valve commissurotomy

- Activity intolerance related to cardiopulmonary dysfunction
- Acute pain related to surgical procedure
- Anxiety related to lack of understanding of procedure
- Decreased cardiac output related to:
  - alterations in afterload
  - alterations in contractility
  - alterations in heart rate or rhythm or both
  - alterations in preload
- Deficient fluid volume related to hypovolemia
- Deficient knowledge related to lack of understanding of procedure and postprocedure care
- Impaired gas exchange related to atelectasis
- Risk for bleeding related to use of anticoagulants
- Risk for infection related to invasive procedure

Heat syndrome

- Deficient knowledge (management of syndrome) related to lack of exposure to information
- Deficient knowledge (prevention) related to language barrier, impaired literacy, or lack of exposure to information
- Hyperthermia related to environmental heat conditions

Hemophilia

- Anxiety related to risk of acute bleeding
- Ineffective protection related to abnormal blood profile
- Risk for injury related to lack of awareness of environmental dangers
- Risk for trauma related to external factors

Hemorrhoids

- Acute pain related to inflammation of hemorrhoidal veins
- Constipation related to pain
- Deficient knowledge related to lack of patient education

Hemothorax

- Acute pain related to blood in pleural cavity
- Anxiety related to acute shortness of breath
- Fear related to sudden onset of injury
- Ineffective breathing pattern related to blood in pleural cavity

Hepatic encephalopathy

- Deficient fluid volume related to edema
- Risk for impaired liver function related to alcohol abuse
- Risk for impaired comfort related to injury, bleeding, or infection
- Risk for injury related to cognitive changes

Hepatitis

- Acute pain related to inflammation of the liver
- Deficient knowledge (home care, disease process, prevention of recurrence) related to lack of exposure to information
- Fatigue related to disease process
- Imbalanced nutrition: Less than body requirements related to anorexia, diarrhea, nausea, or vomiting
- Nausea related to GI irritation
- Risk for activity intolerance related to increased fatigue
- Risk for deficient fluid volume related to vomiting and diarrhea
- Risk for impaired skin integrity related to:
  - frequent diarrhea
  - prolonged bed rest
  - pruritus

Herniated disk

- Activity intolerance related to pain
- Acute pain related to impingement on spinal nerve roots
- Readiness for enhanced management of therapeutic regimen related to ability to follow through with regimen

Herpes simplex

- Acute pain related to cold sores and fever blisters
- Chronic low self-esteem related to skin lesions
- Ineffective sexuality patterns related to fear of spreading infection to sexual partner
- Sexual dysfunction related to sexually transmitted disease (herpes simplex 2)

Herpes zoster

- Acute pain related to inflammation of the dorsal root ganglia
- Chronic pain related to postherpetic neuralgia
- Hyperthermia related to infection
- Impaired skin integrity related to localized vesicular skin lesions

Hiatal hernia

- Acute pain related to displacement of the stomach
- Deficient knowledge (treatment options) related to lack of information
- Impaired swallowing related to esophagitis, ulcers, or strictures
- Risk for aspiration of gastric contents

Hodgkin's disease

- Fatigue related to weight loss and disease process
- Grieving related to perceived potential for loss of life
- Hyperthermia related to immunosuppression
- Ineffective protection related to Hodgkin's disease

Huntington's disease

- Bathing self-care deficit related to physical deterioration
- Bowel incontinence related to neuromuscular impairment
- Caregiver role strain related to complexity and amount of caregiving activities
- Impaired physical mobility related to neuromuscular impairment
- Impaired verbal communication related to dysarthria

Hydronephrosis

- Acute pain related to physical obstruction of urine flow
- Impaired urinary elimination related to obstruction of urine flow
- Risk for infection related to obstruction of urine flow

Hyperaldosteronism

- Deficient knowledge (disease) related to lack of exposure to information
- Fatigue related to hypokalemia
- Impaired urinary elimination related to polyuria and polydipsia
- Risk for unstable glucose level related to hypokalemia

Hyperlipidemia

- Anxiety related to lack of understanding of diagnosis and treatment
- Deficient knowledge related to lack of understanding of diagnosis and treatment
- Fear related to disease prognosis
- Imbalanced nutrition: More than body requirements related to excessive intake of foods high in fat and cholesterol
- Ineffective peripheral tissue perfusion related to buildup of cholesterol in vascular system
- Noncompliance related to failure to adhere to dietary restrictions and medication regimen

- Risk for decreased cardiac tissue perfusion related to narrowing of coronary arteries
- Risk for injury related to disease process

Hyperparathyroidism

- Acute pain related to hypercalcemia, which causes bone tenderness, pancreatitis, and peptic ulcers
- Anxiety related to change in health status and surgical treatment
- Impaired individual resilience related to severity of condition and possibility of a hypercalcemic crisis

Hyperosmolar hyperglycemic nonketotic syndrome

- Deficient fluid volume related to osmotic diuresis
- Deficient knowledge (self-care) related to lack of exposure to complex disease and management
- Risk for injury related to:
  - cerebral dehydration
  - cerebral edema during rapid rehydration
  - decreased perfusion
  - glucose deprivation
  - hypoxemia
- Risk for unstable glucose level related to inadequate insulin secretion or peripheral insulin resistance

Patients with hypertension can be noncompliant as a result of health beliefs or cultural influences.

Hypertension

- Decreased cardiac output related to decreased stroke volume
- Excess fluid volume related to compromised regulatory mechanisms
- Ineffective therapeutic regimen management related to deficient knowledge
- Noncompliance (treatment) related to health beliefs and cultural influences
- Risk for ineffective peripheral tissue perfusion related to decreased blood circulation

Hypoglycemia

- Fatigue related to hypoglycemia
- Ineffective therapeutic regimen management related to complexity of the disease and deficient knowledge
- Risk for injury related to:
  - excessive exercise
  - inappropriate exogenous insulin use
  - lack of food
- errors in medication administration
- financial limitations

Hypoparathyroidism

- Decreased cardiac output related to cardiac arrhythmias
- Imbalanced nutrition: Less than body requirements related to inability to ingest foods due to dysphagia
- Ineffective coping related to situational crisis

Hypothyroidism

- Decreased cardiac output related to cardiac arrhythmias
- Disturbed body image related to periorbital edema and upper eyelid droop
- Risk for dry eye related to reduced quantity or quality of tears to moisten eye
- Risk for imbalanced body temperature related to decreased sensitivity of thermoreceptors

Hypovolemic shock

- Decreased cardiac output related to altered heart rate and rhythm
- Impaired gas exchange related to ventilation-perfusion imbalance
- Ineffective coping related to threat to life
- Ineffective peripheral tissue perfusion related to hypovolemia
- Risk for deficient fluid volume related to:
  - disease processes
  - iatrogenic interventions
  - surgical interventions
- Risk for ineffective cerebral tissue perfusion related to hypovolemia
- Risk for ineffective gastrointestinal perfusion related to hypovolemia
- Risk for ineffective renal perfusion related to hypovolemia
- Risk for injury related to complications from ischemia

Ileal conduit urinary diversion

- Deficient knowledge (care of an ileal conduit) related to lack of exposure to information
- Disturbed body image related to urinary diversion
- Impaired urinary elimination related to creation of an ileal conduit
- Risk for infection related to GI or genitourinary anastomosis breakdown or leakage
- Sexual dysfunction related to cystectomy and possible ejaculatory incompetence with prostatectomy
- Risk for impaired skin integrity related to:
  - sensitive skin around stoma
  - appliance irritation
  - potential for infection

Infertility

- Complicated grieving related to multiple miscarriages
- Ineffective coping related to uncertainty of future pregnancies
- Situational low self-esteem related to infertility

Inflammatory bowel disease

- Chronic pain related to abdominal distention
- Deficient fluid volume related to decreased fluid intake and increased fluid loss through diarrhea
- Imbalanced nutrition: Less than body requirements related to:
  - decreased nutrient intake
  - increased nutrient loss
  - possible decreased bowel absorption
- Impaired skin integrity related to frequent stools and altered nutritional status
- Ineffective sexuality patterns related to diminished physical energy and persistence of uncomfortable physical symptoms
- Insomnia related to:
  - anxiety related to hospitalization
  - nocturnal defecation
  - uncomfortable sensations
- Risk for infection related to:
  - bowel perforation
  - general debilitation
  - immunosuppression
- Social isolation related to dependent behavior

Influenza

- Hyperthermia related to infection
- Ineffective community therapeutic regimen management related to insufficient supply of influenza vaccine
- Risk for imbalanced fluid volume related to fever, cough, decreased oral intake
- Risk for infection related to inadequate primary and secondary defenses to prevent secondary bacterial invasion

Inguinal hernia

- Acute pain related to tension on herniated contents
- Risk for ineffective gastrointestinal perfusion related to diversion of bowel through hernia
- Risk for infection related to complete obstruction

Intestinal obstruction

- Acute pain related to abdominal distention
- Constipation related to intestinal obstruction

- Risk for adverse reaction to iodinated contrast media related to diagnostic procedure
- Risk for deficient fluid volume related to intestinal obstruction
- Risk for dysfunctional gastrointestinal motility
- Risk for ineffective gastrointestinal perfusion related to obstruction

Joint replacement

- Acute pain related to surgery
- Impaired physical mobility related to joint surgery
- Risk for infection related to incision

Kaposi's sarcoma

- Acute pain related to lesions that break down or impinge on nerves and organs
- Grieving related to threat of death in advanced disease and when associated with human immunodeficiency virus
- Impaired skin integrity related to disease process
- Ineffective breathing pattern related to bronchial blockage and hypoventilation

Your patient may have excess fluid volume related to the function of the transplanted kidney. My pail runneth over...

Kidney transplantation

- Acute pain related to frequent invasive procedures and surgery
- Disturbed body image related to effects of steroid therapy
- Excess fluid volume related to function of transplanted kidney
- Ineffective coping related to sensory overload
- Noncompliance (drug regimen) related to adverse drug effects and complicated multidrug regimen
- Risk for infection related to immunosuppression
- Anxiety related to fear of organ rejection and compromised health status

Laminectomy

- Acute pain related to:
  - immobility
  - muscle spasm
  - paresthesia secondary to surgical trauma and postoperative edema
- Deficient knowledge (preoperative and postoperative care) related to lack of exposure to information
- Risk for deficient fluid volume related to:
  - blood loss during surgery
  - hemorrhage at the incision site
  - retroperitoneal hemorrhage
  - vascular injury

- Risk for ineffective renal tissue perfusion related to:
  - anesthesia
  - anxiety
  - cord edema
  - injury to the spinal nerve roots innervating the bladder
  - opioids
  - pain
  - supine positioning

Laryngeal cancer
- Acute pain related to drinking citrus or hot liquid or tumor pressure
- Imbalanced nutrition: Less than body requirements related to impaired swallowing
- Impaired swallowing related to tumor
- Impaired verbal communication related to laryngectomy
- Disturbed body image related to neck surgery and altered appearance

Legionnaires' disease
- Diarrhea related to infection
- Fatigue related to infection
- Hyperthermia related to infection
- Ineffective airway clearance related to increased mucus production
- Risk for infection related to inadequate immune defenses to prevent secondary bacterial invasion

Leukemia
- Activity intolerance related to:
  - depressed nutritional status
  - fatigue secondary to rapid destruction of leukemic cells
  - tissue hypoxia secondary to anemia
- Acute pain related to physical, biological, or chemical agents
- Deficient knowledge (therapeutic modality and choice and care of vascular access device) related to lack of exposure to information
- Fatigue related to rapid destruction of leukemic cells
- Hopelessness related to prognosis
- Imbalanced nutrition: Less than body requirements related to:
  - anorexia
  - chemotherapy
  - nausea
  - taste perception changes
  - vomiting
- Impaired oral mucous membrane related to:
  - cytotoxic effects of chemotherapy
  - immunosuppression secondary to disease

- Ineffective coping related to uncertain prognosis and multiple disease- and treatment-induced losses
- Ineffective protection related to severe immunosuppression associated with bone marrow transplantation or peripheral stem cell transplantation protocol
- Readiness for enhanced immunization status related to successful bone marrow transplantation
- Risk for deficient fluid volume related to risk of hemorrhage
- Risk for infection related to immunosuppression

Liver abscess

- Acute pain related to liver abscess
- Anxiety related to change in health status
- Impaired gas exchange related to abnormal breathing rate and rhythm due to pain
- Risk for imbalanced body temperature related to infection

Liver failure

- Imbalanced nutrition: Less than body requirements related to catabolism caused by liver disease
- Impaired skin integrity related to:
  - ascites
  - increased bleeding tendencies
  - jaundice
  - malnutrition
- Risk for acute confusion related to hepatic encephalopathy syndrome
- Risk for imbalanced fluid volume related to ascites
- Risk for infection related to liver disease

Remember that every patient may have different needs. The nursing diagnoses listed here are those that are most commonly associated with each medical condition.

Liver transplantation

- Acute pain related to surgery
- Compromised family coping related to prolonged disease
- Imbalanced nutrition: Less than body requirements related to:
  - anorexia
  - chronic illness
  - initial postoperative nothing-by-mouth status
- Ineffective breathing pattern related to prolonged general anesthesia and a large abdominal incision
- Readiness for enhanced hope related to new liver
- Risk for deficient fluid volume related to high-dose steroid therapy and fluid loss
- Risk for impaired liver function related to surgery and disease process
- Risk for infection related to surgical incision and immunosuppression

Lung abscess
- Hyperthermia related to infection
- Impaired gas exchange related to altered oxygen supply
- Ineffective airway clearance related to increased secretions

Lung cancer
- Activity intolerance related to imbalance between oxygen supply and demand
- Imbalanced nutrition: Less than body requirements related to inability to ingest food
- Ineffective airway clearance related to excessive secretions and fatigue
- Powerlessness related to perceived mortality
- Risk for adverse reaction to iodinated contrast media related to diagnostic procedure
- Fatigue related to pain, lack of sleep, treatments, poor nutrition, and the stress of the disease process

Lupus erythematosus
- Decreased cardiac output related to pericarditis, myocarditis, or endocarditis
- Hyperthermia related to immunosuppression
- Impaired physical mobility related to joint inflammation
- Impaired skin integrity related to rashes
- Risk-prone health behavior related to disability

Lyme disease
- Acute pain related to arthritis
- Anxiety related to long treatment course
- Fatigue related to infection
- Impaired skin integrity related to rash

Lymphoma, non-Hodgkin's
- Anxiety related to unknown hospital procedures and threat to health status
- Deficient knowledge (self-care of vascular access device, including peripherally or centrally inserted venous catheters or subcutaneous ports) related to lack of exposure to information
- Disturbed body image related to effects of chemotherapy or radiation therapy
- Imbalanced nutrition: Less than body requirements related to:
  - altered oral mucous membrane
  - anorexia
  - fatigue
  - nausea and vomiting
  - taste alterations

- Impaired skin integrity related to effects of radiation therapy
- Ineffective protection related to immunosuppression
- Risk for infection related to:
  - chemotherapy
  - leukopenia, lymphopenia from bone marrow involvement
  - radiation therapy effects

Macular degeneration

- Impaired physical mobility related to vision impairment
- Powerlessness related to illness progression

Malignant melanoma

- Disturbed body image related to skin lesion on head or neck
- Impaired skin integrity related to sore, inflamed, itchy skin lesion
- Readiness for enhanced management of therapeutic regimen related to understanding treatment protocols

Mastectomy

- Anxiety related to fear of cancer recurrence
- Deficient knowledge (treatment options) related to lack of exposure to information
- Disturbed body image related to loss of a body part
- Risk for infection related to incision
- Grieving related to loss of breast
- Impaired physical mobility related to lymph node, muscle, or nerve damage and pain

Maze procedure for atrial fibrillation

- Activity intolerance related to cardiopulmonary dysfunction
- Anxiety related to lack of understanding of surgical procedure
- Decreased cardiac output related to alteration in hemodynamic status
- Deficient fluid volume related to hypovolemia
- Deficient knowledge related to lack of understanding of procedure
- Fear related to lack of understanding of surgical procedure
- Risk for infection related to invasive procedure

Mechanical ventilation

- Bathing self-care deficit related to impaired mobility status and pain
- Deficient fluid volume related to:
  - altered oral intake
  - fluid retention
  - osmotic diuresis
- Deficient knowledge (peripheral parenteral nutrition [PPN] catheter care and therapy) related to lack of experience with PPN

- Fear related to inability to speak and dependence on life support
- Imbalanced nutrition: Less than body requirements related to inability to ingest nutrients orally or digest them satisfactorily, or to increased need
- Impaired bed mobility related to ventilator
- Impaired gas exchange related to insufficient oxygen levels
- Ineffective airway clearance related to:
  - ○ increased secretions
  - ○ presence of an endotracheal tube
  - ○ underlying disease
- Risk for dry eye related to reduced quantity or quality of tears to moisten eye.
- Risk for impaired skin integrity related to physical immobility
- Risk for infection related to central venous catheter
- Risk for injury related to:
  - ○ bypassed safety alarm mechanisms
  - ○ complications of PPN catheter insertion
  - ○ increased intrathoracic pressure
  - ○ mechanical breakdown
  - ○ patient deterioration

Ménière's disease

- Deficient knowledge (symptom prevention and control measures) related to recent onset of disease
- Impaired physical mobility related to vertigo
- Risk for falls related to vertigo
- Sedentary lifestyle related to vertigo

Meningitis

- Acute pain related to headache, joint involvement, or muscle aches from infection
- Hyperthermia related to infection
- Risk for ineffective cerebral tissue perfusion related to increased intracranial pressure
- Risk for injury related to seizures

Metabolic acidosis

- Deficient fluid volume related to active loss from diarrhea and vomiting
- Ineffective breathing pattern related to fatigue and Kussmaul's respirations
- Nausea related to GI distress

Metabolic alkalosis

- Ineffective breathing pattern related to hypoventilation
- Risk for injury related to muscle weakness

Multiple myeloma

- Acute pain related to neoplasm that infiltrates the bone
- Fatigue related to illness
- Risk for infection related to immunosuppression

Multiple sclerosis

- Compromised family coping related to effects of progressive, debilitating disease on family members and resultant alteration in role-related behavior patterns
- Constipation related to decreased peristalsis
- Dressing/grooming self-care deficit related to neuromuscular impairment
- Fatigue related to weakness and spasticity
- Impaired physical mobility related to demyelinization
- Impaired verbal communication related to dysarthria
- Interrupted family processes related to role disturbance and uncertain future
- Powerlessness related to remissions and exacerbations of illness
- Readiness for enhanced comfort related to acceptance of care and support of significant others
- Risk for caregiver role strain related to progressive debilitating disease
- Risk for injury related to:
  - gait impairment
  - vertigo
  - vision disturbances
- Risk for thermal injury related to neuromuscular impairment
- Sexual dysfunction related to fatigue, decreased sensation, muscle spasm, or urinary incontinence
- Situational low self-esteem related to progressive, debilitating effects of disease
- Urinary retention related to sensorimotor deficits

Myasthenia gravis

- Activity intolerance related to muscle fatigue and weakness
- Dressing self-care deficit related to neuromuscular involvement
- Fatigue related to muscle weakness
- Impaired swallowing related to cerebellar dysfunction
- Ineffective airway clearance related to impaired ability to cough
- Ineffective therapeutic regimen management related to insufficient knowledge of disease and medication usage
- Risk for injury related to vision disturbance and weakness
- Risk for spiritual distress related to chronic illness
- Risk for urge urinary incontinence related to neuromuscular involvement

Says here that patients can experience death anxiety related to a diagnosis of myocardial infarction. Yikes!

Myocardial infarction

- Activity intolerance related to weakness and fatigue
- Acute pain (chest) related to decreased myocardial oxygenation
- Death anxiety related to diagnosis
- Decreased cardiac output related to altered heart rate or rhythm
- Deficient knowledge (diagnostic procedures, therapeutic interventions, and long-range implications for lifestyle changes) related to complex diagnosis and therapeutic regimen
- Impaired gas exchange related to ventilation-perfusion imbalance
- Ineffective coping related to fear of death, anxiety, denial, or depression
- Risk for adverse reaction to iodinated contrast media related to diagnostic procedure
- Risk for constipation related to diet, bed rest, or medications
- Risk for injury related to myocardial ischemia, injury, necrosis, inflammation, or arrhythmias
- Risk for ineffective peripheral tissue perfusion related to decreased blood circulation

Myocarditis

- Activity intolerance related to weakness and fatigue
- Decreased cardiac output related to arrhythmias
- Fatigue related to infection

Nephrectomy

- Acute pain related to surgical procedure
- Ineffective airway clearance related to:
  - anesthesia
  - immobility
  - location of incision
  - pain
  - presence of chest tube
- Risk for imbalanced fluid volume related to decreased renal reserve and third-space fluid shifting immediately after surgery
- Risk for perioperative positioning related to flank positioning and outermost arm positioning
- Ineffective coping related to fear and anxiety about disease process

Nephrotic syndrome

- Imbalanced nutrition: Less than body requirements related to high-protein, low-sodium diet
- Risk for imbalanced fluid volume related to disease process
- Risk for infection related to immunosuppression
- Deficient knowledge (symptoms of disease progression, medications, diet recommendations, and home care) related to lack of information

Neuritis, peripheral
- Impaired physical mobility related to muscle weakness
- Risk for injury related to disturbed sensory perception

Neurogenic bladder
- Reflex urinary incontinence related to neuromuscular dysfunction of the lower urinary tract
- Risk for compromised human dignity related to incontinence
- Risk for infection related to incomplete emptying of bladder
- Risk for urinary incontinence related to neuromuscular dysfunction

Obesity
- Activity intolerance related to deconditioned status and excessive energy demands secondary to obesity
- Disturbed body image related to social stigma of obesity
- Imbalanced nutrition: More than body requirements related to:
  - dysfunctional eating patterns
  - energy expenditure imbalance
  - excess food intake
  - inherited disposition
  - sedentary activity level
- Impaired gas exchange related to ventilation-perfusion imbalance
- Impaired physical mobility related to fatigue with minimal exertion, joint or back discomfort, limitation of motion from extra skin folds
- Risk for impaired skin integrity related to:
  - altered circulation (edema)
  - multiple moist skin folds
  - nutritional deficit
- Risk for ineffective peripheral tissue perfusion related to decreased blood circulation
- Sedentary lifestyle related to weight
- Social isolation related to size too large for standard seating and body image disturbance
- Ineffective coping related to using food inappropriately to comfort self when anxious, distressed, or traumatized

Osteoarthritis
- Activity intolerance related to pain
- Chronic pain related to deterioration of joint cartilage
- Impaired home maintenance related to inadequate support systems or decreased range of motion with increased joint pain

Osteomyelitis

- Acute pain related to inflammation
- Deficient knowledge (prolonged treatment regimen for infection and measures to prevent recurrence) related to new diagnosis
- Impaired physical mobility related to pain
- Risk for disuse syndrome related to prolonged infection, pain, and immobilization
- Risk for injury related to use of antibiotics with high potential for toxic effects

Osteoporosis

- Anxiety related to change in health status and mobility limitations
- Disturbed body image related to joint deformity
- Ineffective sexuality patterns related to pain
- Risk for adverse reaction to iodinated contrast media related to diagnostic procedure
- Risk for dry eye related to reduced quantity or quality of tears to moisten eye
- Risk for trauma related to bone loss

Otosclerosis

- Deficient knowledge (disease) related to lack of exposure to information
- Risk for infection related to surgery

Ovarian cancer

- Constipation related to GI obstruction
- Deficient knowledge (disease and treatment options) related to lack of exposure to information
- Grieving related to loss of fertility
- Urinary retention related to obstruction

Ovarian cyst

- Acute pain related to complications of ovarian cysts that cause acute abdominal symptoms
- Anxiety related to laparoscopic surgery
- Ineffective sexuality patterns related to irregular or prolonged bleeding

Paget's disease

- Acute pain related to impingement of abnormal bone on spinal cord
- Bathing, dressing, toileting self-care deficit related to musculoskeletal impairment

- Disturbed body image related to musculoskeletal impairment
- Impaired physical mobility related to asymmetrical bowing of tibia and femur

Pancreatic cancer

- Acute pain related to tumor pressure
- Anxiety related to threat of death and disease status
- Caregiver role strain related to illness severity
- Imbalanced nutrition: Less than body requirements related to:
  - impaired digestion
  - loss of appetite
  - pain
  - vomiting
- Risk for adverse reaction to iodinated contrast media related to diagnostic procedure

Pancreatitis

- Acute pain related to:
  - abscess formation or hemorrhaging
  - autodigestive processes and necrosis
  - edema of the pancreas and surrounding tissues
  - peritonitis
- Imbalanced nutrition: Less than body requirements related to:
  - gastric suction
  - impaired digestion
  - nothing-by-mouth status
  - vomiting
- Nausea related to gastric distention
- Risk for deficient fluid volume related to:
  - fluid shifts
  - hemorrhage
  - hyperglycemia
  - vomiting
- Risk for infection related to trauma and chronic disease
- Risk for injury related to:
  - alcoholism
  - hypovolemia
  - pulmonary insults
  - Ineffective breathing pattern related to secretions, pulmonary infiltrates, atelectasis, and pain

Watch patients with pancreatitis for signs of imbalanced nutrition. I'm feeling queasy just looking at this list.

Parkinson's disease

- Activity intolerance related to neuromuscular impairment
- Bathing self-care deficit related to neuromuscular impairment
- Disturbed body image related to tremors
- Impaired home maintenance related to disease effects

- Risk for aspiration related to impaired muscles of swallowing
- Risk for falls related to impaired gait and balance
- Sedentary lifestyle related to neuromuscular impairment

Pelvic inflammatory disease
- Acute pain related to inflammation
- Risk for infection related to inadequate primary defenses
- Sexual dysfunction related to malaise and profuse, purulent vaginal discharge

Peptic ulcers
- Acute pain related to ulcers
- Deficient knowledge (ulcer prevention and care) related to lack of exposure to information
- Nausea related to GI distress

Percutaneous transluminal coronary angioplasty
- Acute pain related to restrictions on mobility and percutaneous puncture at groin site
- Anxiety related to known risks associated with the procedure
- Deficient knowledge (postdischarge care) related to lack of exposure to information
- Risk for adverse reaction to iodinated contrast media related to diagnostic procedure
- Risk for injury related to break in skin and presence of foreign body intravascularly

Pericarditis
- Acute pain related to inflammation of pericardium
- Decreased cardiac output related to pericarditis
- Risk for decreased cardiac tissue perfusion related to decreased cellular exchange
- Deficient knowledge (home care, disease process) related to lack of information

Peripheral vascular disease
- Activity intolerance related to pain
- Impaired physical mobility related to pain and activity intolerance
- Ineffective peripheral tissue perfusion related to decreased oxygenation
- Risk for peripheral neurovascular dysfunction related to vascular obstruction

Perirectal abscess and fistula
- Acute pain related to abscess and fistula
- Delayed surgical recovery related to inflammation and infection
- Situational low self-esteem related to difficult healing process

Peritonitis

- Acute pain related to inflammation
- Nausea related to increased GI pressure
- Risk for infection related to inadequate primary defenses

Permanent pacemaker insertion

- Bathing self-care deficit related to bed rest and activity limitations
- Deficient knowledge (self-care after discharge) related to unfamiliar therapeutic intervention
- Disturbed body image related to dependence on pacemaker
- Risk for infection related to surgical disruption of skin barrier

Pituitary tumor

- Acute pain related to tumor pressure
- Deficient knowledge (surgical options) related to lack of exposure to information
- Disturbed sensory perception (visual) related to unilateral blindness
- Risk for injury related to dementia

Pleural effusion and empyema

- Fatigue related to weakness, dyspnea, cough, and anorexia
- Hyperthermia related to infection
- Ineffective breathing pattern related to pain and increased work of breathing

Pleurisy

- Acute pain related to inflammation of visceral and parietal pleurae
- Impaired gas exchange related to altered oxygen supply
- Ineffective breathing pattern related to limited movement on affected side

Pneumocystis jiroveci (carinii) pneumonia

- Fatigue related to infection, compromised nutrition, and depression
- Grieving related to poor prognosis
- Ineffective breathing pattern related to fatigue
- Risk for imbalanced body temperature related to infection

Pneumonia

- Acute pain related to fever and pleuritic irritation
- Bathing/hygiene self-care deficit related to weakness and fatigue
- Deficient fluid volume related to active fluid volume loss
- Deficient knowledge (treatment regimen) related to lack of exposure to information

- Impaired gas exchange related to ventilation-perfusion imbalance
- Ineffective airway clearance related to retained secretions
- Risk for infection related to stress and other risk factors

Pneumonectomy

- Acute pain related to surgical procedure
- Anxiety related to breathing difficulty
- Anxiety related to lack of understanding of diagnosis and treatment
- Deficient knowledge related to lack of understanding of surgical procedure and prognosis
- Disturbed body image related to change in body function
- Fear related to lack of understanding of diagnosis and treatment
- Impaired gas exchange related to alveolar hypoventilation
- Impaired physical mobility related to pain from surgical procedure
- Ineffective airway clearance related to inadequate pain control and splinting of surgical site to promote effective coughing and deep breathing
- Ineffective breathing pattern related to decreased lung expansion
- Risk for infection related to surgical procedure

Pneumothorax

- Acute pain related to air trapped in the intrapleural space
- Fear related to sudden onset of illness
- Impaired gas exchange related to ventilation-perfusion imbalance
- Ineffective tissue perfusion (cardiopulmonary) related to collapsed lung
- Anxiety related to breathing difficulty

Polycystic kidney disease

- Acute pain related to kidney mass
- Deficient knowledge (illness) related to lack of exposure to information
- Risk for ineffective renal perfusion related to kidney mass

Polycythemia vera

- Acute pain related to headache
- Deficient knowledge (disease and treatment) related to lack of exposure to information
- Impaired gas exchange related to dyspnea

Potassium imbalance

- Decreased cardiac output related to arrhythmias
- Diarrhea related to hypercalcemia and hypocalcemia
- Nausea related to GI distress

Lack of exposure to information can lead to deficient knowledge about an illness. I thought I might do a little reading about polycystic kidney disease.

Pressure ulcers

- Imbalanced nutrition: Less than body requirements related to inability to digest and absorb nutrients
- Impaired physical mobility related to musculoskeletal and neuro-muscular impairment
- Impaired skin integrity related to:
  - altered circulation
  - altered sensation
  - impaired physical mobility
  - mechanical factors
- Risk for infection related to impaired skin integrity

Prostatectomy

- Acute pain related to:
  - bladder spasms
  - catheter obstruction
  - surgical intervention
  - urethral stricture
- Risk for deficient fluid volume related to prostatic or incisional bleeding after surgery
- Risk for infection (postoperative) related to:
  - abdominal drain placement
  - preoperative status
  - urinary catheter
- Risk for situational low self-esteem related to:
  - incontinence
  - potential impotence
  - sexual alterations
- Sexual dysfunction (decreased libido) related to:
  - decreased self-esteem
  - fear of incontinence
  - impotence related to parasympathetic nerve damage (from radical prostatectomy)
  - infertility related to retrograde ejaculation (from transurethral resection of the prostate and suprapubic prostatectomy)
- Urge urinary incontinence related to:
  - decrease in detrusor muscle
  - sphincter tone
  - trauma to the bladder neck
  - urinary catheter removal
- Urinary retention related to urinary catheter obstruction

Prostatic cancer

- Acute pain related to physical, biological, or chemical agents
- Anxiety related to change in health status
- Sexual dysfunction related to impotence
- Urinary retention related to obstruction and infection

Prostatitis

- Acute pain related to infection and difficulty to urinate
- Hyperthermia related to infection
- Impaired urinary elimination related to infection

Pseudomembranous enterocolitis

- Deficient fluid volume related to active loss
- Diarrhea related to inflammation
- Impaired skin integrity related to severe diarrhea

Psoriasis

- Disturbed body image related to itchy, dry, cracked, and encrusted lesions on body parts
- Impaired skin integrity related to itchy, dry, cracked, and encrusted lesions
- Social isolation related to disturbed body image

Pulmonary edema

- Decreased cardiac output related to tachycardia
- Dysfunctional ventilatory weaning response related to anxiety
- Excess fluid volume related to fluid accumulation in extravascular spaces of the lungs
- Ineffective breathing pattern related to diminished lung compliance

Pulmonary embolism and infarction

- Activity intolerance related to imbalance between oxygen supply and demand
- Acute pain related to biological injury
- Compromised family coping related to potentially life-threatening situation
- Decreased cardiac output related to altered heart rate and rhythm
- Deficient fluid volume related to active fluid volume loss
- Deficient knowledge (treatment regimen) related to complex disorder and therapy
- Impaired gas exchange related to ventilation-perfusion imbalance

Pulmonary hypertension

- Bathing self-care deficit related to fatigue
- Decreased cardiac output related to altered heart rate and rhythm
- Ineffective breathing pattern related to hypertrophy of small pulmonary arteries
- Risk for decreased cardiac tissue perfusion related to impaired transport of oxygen across alveolocapillary membranes

Pyelonephritis

- Excess fluid volume related to compromised regulatory mechanisms
- Hyperthermia related to infection
- Impaired urinary elimination related to urgency, burning, or nocturia
- Risk for infection related to inadequate primary and secondary defenses

Radioactive implant for cervical cancer

- Ineffective sexuality patterns related to vaginal tissue changes or fear of radioactivity
- Risk for disuse syndrome related to imposed bed rest
- Risk for injury related to dislodgment of the implant

Rape trauma syndrome

- Rape trauma syndrome related to rape or attempted rape and psychological response
- Situational low self-esteem related to rape

Raynaud's disease

- Ineffective peripheral tissue perfusion related to decreased arterial blood flow
- Risk for impaired skin integrity related to decreased sensation and ischemia

Renal calculi

- Acute pain related to obstruction of ureter or kidney by renal calculi
- Deficient knowledge (disease) related to lack of exposure to information
- Risk for infection related to trauma
- Urinary retention related to ureter obstruction by renal calculi

Renal dialysis

- Acute pain related to hemodialysis treatment
- Imbalanced nutrition: Less than body requirements related to:
  - abdominal distention
  - anorexia
  - nausea
  - stomatitis
- Impaired physical mobility related to lengthy treatment regimen and fatigue
- Ineffective breathing pattern related to elevation of diaphragm during peritoneal dialysis exchanges and reduced mobility

Patients with Raynaud's disease are at risk for impaired skin integrity related to decreased sensation. Is it cold in here, or is it just me?

- Risk for acute confusion related to consequences of long-term dialysis treatment
- Risk for fluid imbalance related to dialysis
- Risk for infection related to invasive procedure
- Risk for injury related to:
  - bleeding from the area around the vascular access device
  - potential for thrombosis, stenosis, or hematoma of vascular access
- Risk for injury (perforation or ileus) related to catheter insertion or irritation from dialysate

Renal failure, acute

- Deficient knowledge (acute renal failure and dialysis) related to lack of exposure to information on complex disease and its management
- Excess fluid volume related to sodium and water retention
- Imbalanced nutrition: Less than body requirements related to anorexia, nausea and vomiting, and restricted dietary intake
- Impaired urinary elimination related to disease process
- Risk for infection related to decreased immune response and skin changes secondary to uremia
- Risk for injury related to uremic syndrome

Renal failure, chronic

- Caregiver role strain related to illness chronicity
- Chronic low self-esteem related to chronic disease and depression
- Disturbed thought processes related to:
  - acidosis
  - fluid and electrolyte imbalances
  - uremic toxins
- Excess fluid volume related to fluid retention
- Imbalanced nutrition: Less than body requirements related to:
  - altered metabolism of proteins, lipids, and carbohydrates
  - anorexia
  - diarrhea
  - GI inflammation with poor absorption
  - nausea and vomiting
  - restricted dietary intake
- Impaired oral mucous membrane related to accumulation of urea and ammonia
- Noncompliance (treatment regimen) related to:
  - deficient knowledge
  - denial
  - lack of resources
  - lack of social support systems

- Risk for impaired skin integrity related to:
  - abnormal blood clotting
  - anemia
  - calcium phosphate deposits on the skin
  - capillary fragility
  - decreased activity of oil and sweat glands
  - retention of pigments
  - scratching
- Sexual dysfunction related to the effects of uremia on the endocrine system and central nervous system and to the psychosocial impact of chronic renal failure and its treatment

Respiratory acidosis

- Decreased cardiac output related to altered heart rate and rhythm
- Impaired gas exchange related to ventilatory-perfusion imbalance
- Ineffective breathing pattern related to hypoventilation

Respiratory alkalosis

- Anxiety related to hyperventilation
- Impaired gas exchange related to ventilatory-perfusion imbalance
- Ineffective breathing pattern related to hyperventilation

Retinal detachment

- Impaired physical mobility related to vision disturbance
- Ineffective coping related to decreased vision and impending surgery and fear of postoperative complications
- Risk for falls related to impaired vision

Rheumatoid arthritis

- Activity intolerance related to pain and swelling of joints
- Chronic pain related to inflammation of joints
- Disturbed body image related to arthritic joints
- Ineffective health maintenance related to lack of mobility
- Risk for dry eye related to reduced quantity or quality of tears to moisten the eye

Rhinoplasty

- Acute pain related to surgical manipulation and swelling
- Anxiety related to lack of understanding of surgical procedure and self-care after surgery
- Deficient knowledge related to lack of understanding of what is involved in surgical procedure
- Disturbed sleep pattern related to pain and edema
- Fear related to surgical procedure

- Impaired skin integrity related to surgical intervention
- Ineffective breathing pattern related to nasal packing
- Risk for infection related to surgical procedure
- Risk for injury related to tissue trauma

Salmonellosis

- Diarrhea related to GI distress
- Hyperthermia related to infection
- Risk for deficient fluid volume related to diarrhea

Sarcoidosis

- Activity intolerance related to pain
- Decreased cardiac output related to arrhythmias
- Deficient knowledge (disease and treatment) related to lack of information about the disease and medication
- Ineffective breathing pattern related to pain

Scabies

- Impaired skin integrity related to skin infection
- Ineffective sexual patterns related to fear of spreading infection
- Social isolation related to fear of spreading infection

Seizure disorder

- Acute confusion related to postictal state
- Deficient knowledge (seizure management) related to lack of exposure to information
- Impaired memory related to neurologic disturbance
- Ineffective airway clearance related to:
  - airway occlusion by tongue or foreign body
  - apnea
  - excessive secretions
  - jaw clenching
  - loss of consciousness
- Ineffective therapeutic regimen management related to deficient knowledge of disease, seizure care, and community resources
- Risk for injury related to excessive uncontrolled muscle activity
- Risk for trauma related to internal and external factors

Septic arthritis

- Acute pain related to inflammation of joints, open wounds, or postoperative complications
- Anxiety related to threat to health and roles
- Risk for infection related to inadequate primary and secondary defenses

Septic shock

- Acute confusion related to decreased cerebral tissue perfusion
- Diarrhea related to GI irritation
- Hyperthermia related to infection
- Imbalanced nutrition: Less than body requirements related to inadequate intake and active fluid and nutrient loss
- Impaired gas exchange related to ventilation-perfusion imbalance and diffusion defects
- Ineffective coping related to threat to life
- Risk for injury due to complications related to ischemia or bleeding

Sinusitis

- Acute pain related to inflammation and pressure
- Fatigue related to infection and headache
- Risk for infection related to inadequate primary defenses

Sjögren's syndrome

- Fatigue related to disease process
- Impaired oral mucous membrane related to oral dryness
- Deficient knowledge (symptoms of disease management, self-care, and treatment options) related to lack of exposure to information

Skin grafts

- Deficient knowledge (home care of donor and graft sites) related to lack of exposure to information
- Disturbed body image related to wound and potential scarring
- Imbalanced nutrition: Less than body requirements related to increased metabolic needs secondary to tissue healing
- Impaired physical mobility related to position and movement limitations
- Risk for infection of donor site related to surgical excision

Spinal cord injury

- Bathing self-care deficit related to spinal cord injury
- Constipation related to loss of voluntary bowel control
- Decreased cardiac output related to autonomic dysfunction and immobility
- Deficient diversional activity related to loss of mobility or function
- Disturbed body image related to physical disability
- Imbalanced nutrition: Less than body requirements related to acute injury
- Impaired gas exchange related to loss of use of phrenic nerve, intercostal muscles, or abdominal muscles secondary to the spinal injury

- Impaired home maintenance related to inadequate support systems
- Impaired physical mobility related to muscle paralysis
- Impaired urinary elimination related to interruption of neural innervation
- Incontinence, bowel and total urinary related to neuromuscular enervation
- Ineffective airway clearance related to loss of use of intercostal muscles
- Risk for autonomic dysreflexia related to damage to spinal cord with another associated stressor
- Risk for infection related to catheterization

Spinal cord injuries can cause many problems not the least of which is a deficit related to self-care. Brush up on the ones listed here.

Spinal neoplasm

- Impaired physical mobility related to neuromuscular impairment
- Incontinence, bowel and total urinary related to neurologic dysfunction
- Risk for autonomic dysreflexia related to spinal cord injury or lesion
- Risk for impaired skin integrity related to:
  - altered nutritional status
  - altered sensation
  - mechanical factors
  - moisture from incontinence
  - physical immobilization

Squamous cell carcinoma

- Anxiety related to threat to health status
- Impaired skin integrity related to invasive tumor of skin
- Ineffective therapeutic regimen management related to deficient knowledge

Stomatitis

- Acute pain related to swollen and easily bruised gums and mucous membranes
- Imbalanced nutrition: Less than body requirements related to presence of oral lesions
- Impaired oral mucous membrane related to:
  - chemical irritants
  - infection
  - malnutrition or vitamin deficiency
  - mechanical irritants (ill-fitting dentures, braces)
- Risk for infection related to immunosuppression
- Risk for infection related to radiation or chemotherapy treatment and immunosuppression

Stroke

- Bathing self-care deficit related to:
    - neuromuscular impairment
    - perceptual cognitive impairment
    - weakness or lack of motivation
- Caregiver role strain related to increased care needs
- Chronic confusion related to cerebral injury
- Deficient knowledge (stroke management) related to lack of exposure to information on self-care
- Impaired physical mobility related to damage to motor cortex or motor pathways
- Impaired verbal communication related to cerebral injury
- Ineffective airway clearance related to hemiplegic effects of a stroke
- Risk for adverse reaction to iodinated contrast media related to diagnostic procedure
- Risk for disuse syndrome related to neuromuscular impairment
- Risk for ineffective cerebral tissue perfusion related to clot or hemorrhage
- Risk for thermal injury related to neuromuscular impairment
- Unilateral neglect related to cerebral injury
- Ineffective coping related to neurological deficits, depression, mobility issues, alterations in performing self-care and participating in diversional activities

Syphilis

- Ineffective coping related to situational crisis, threatened relationship, and stigma
- Ineffective sexuality patterns related to fear of spreading illness
- Risk for infection related to external factors

Tendinitis and bursitis

- Activity intolerance related to pain and stiffness
- Acute pain related to inflammation
- Ineffective role performance related to restricted movement of joint due to pain

Thoracotomy

- Acute pain related to surgical incision
- Deficient knowledge (treatment regimen) related to unfamiliarity with thoracotomy and postoperative treatment and home care
- Impaired gas exchange related to:
    - analgesic medications
    - atelectasis
    - hypoventilation from anesthesia
    - pain
    - thickened secretions

- Risk for infection related to surgical incision and endotracheal intubation

Thrombocytopenia
- Decreased cardiac output related to tachycardia
- Deficient knowledge (disease and treatment) related to lack of exposure to information particularly related to patient safety
- Fatigue related to disease process
- Risk for injury related to possible bleeding from lack of platelets

Thrombophlebitis
- Acute pain related to vessel obstruction and edema
- Deficient knowledge (treatment regimen) related to lack of exposure to information
- Ineffective peripheral tissue perfusion related to interruption of venous flow

Thyroid cancer
- Deficient knowledge (treatment regimen) related to lack of exposure to information
- Impaired swallowing related to pressure of thyroid nodule
- Ineffective breathing pattern related to enlarged thyroid nodule
- Risk for adverse reaction to iodinated contrast media related to diagnostic procedure

Toxic shock syndrome
- Diarrhea related to infection
- Fear related to sudden onset of illness and complications
- Hyperthermia related to infection

Tracheostomy
- Impaired skin integrity related to humidity, moisture, or mucus accumulation
- Ineffective breathing pattern related to tracheal tube dislodgment or plugging
- Risk for aspiration related to impaired swallowing and vomiting
- Risk for injury (poor oxygenation) related to suctioning procedure

Transcranial magnetic stimulation
- Acute pain related to stimulation of cranial nerves
- Anxiety related to lack of understanding of procedure
- Deficient knowledge related to lack of understanding of process or procedure and possible outcomes
- Fear related to lack of understanding of procedure
- Impaired skin integrity related to burns from electrode heating
- Risk for injury related to possible seizure activity

Trauma

- Impaired gas exchange related to:
  - ○ head injury
  - ○ pulmonary injury
  - ○ shock
- Impaired physical mobility related to orthopedic injury
- Risk for imbalanced fluid volume related to hypovolemia or cardiac injury
- Risk for injury (complications) related to:
  - ○ hypermetabolic state
  - ○ impaired immunologic defenses
  - ○ stress
- Risk for posttrauma syndrome related to perception of event and sudden, unexpected injury

Trigeminal neuralgia

- Acute pain related to disorder of the fifth cranial nerve
- Anxiety related to threat to health
- Ineffective coping related to inadequate level of perception of control of factors that aggravate pain

Trigeminal neuralgia can cause acute pain. What nerve!

Tuberculosis

- Deficient knowledge (disease process) related to lack of exposure to information
- Ineffective airway clearance related to tracheobronchial obstruction or secretions
- Ineffective breathing pattern related to decreased energy or fatigue
- Risk for infection related to altered primary defenses
- Social isolation related to fear of spreading disease

Ulcerative colitis

- Anxiety related to change in health status
- Diarrhea related to inflammation of colon
- Fatigue related to loss of fluids and diarrhea
- Imbalanced nutrition: Less than body requirements related to inability to absorb nutrients
- Ineffective role performance related to frequent diarrhea

Urinary tract infection

- Acute pain related to inflammation and muscle spasms
- Deficient knowledge (disease process) related to lack of exposure to information
- Impaired urinary elimination related to obstruction

Urolithiasis

- Acute pain related to:
    - incision
    - passage of calculus fragments
    - procedural manipulation
- Deficient knowledge (potential causes of calculus formation) related to lack of exposure to information
- Impaired urinary elimination: Dysuria, oliguria, pyuria, or frequency related to:
    - calculus fragment passage
    - hematuria
    - infection
    - obstruction

Uterine cancer

- Acute pain related to cancer
- Imbalanced nutrition: Less than body requirements related to cancer
- Risk for adverse reaction to iodinated contrast media related to diagnostic procedure
- Spiritual distress related to chronic illness and loss of fertility

Uterine prolapse

- Anxiety related to change in health status
- Disturbed body image related to biophysical factors
- Stress urinary incontinence related to weak pelvic musculature

Valvular heart disease

- Activity intolerance related to fatigue and dyspnea on exertion
- Anxiety related to change in health status
- Decreased cardiac output related to mechanical disruption
- Ineffective breathing pattern related to decreased energy and fatigue

Vascular retinopathy

- Ineffective coping related to chronic illness
- Risk for injury related to loss of vision

Vasculitis

- Disturbed body image related to illness
- Imbalanced nutrition: Less than body requirements related to anorexia of disease process
- Ineffective peripheral tissue perfusion related to inflamed vessels causing impaired blood flow to nearby organs

- Risk for ineffective cerebral tissue perfusion related to inflamed vessels causing impaired blood flow to nearby organs
- Risk for ineffective gastrointestinal perfusion related to inflamed vessels causing impaired blood flow to nearby organs
- Risk for ineffective renal perfusion related to inflamed vessels causing impaired blood flow to nearby organs
- Risk for infection related to impaired defenses

Vulvovaginitis

- Acute pain related to inflammation
- Ineffective sexuality patterns related to vaginal inflammation, itching, and irritation
- Risk for infection related to inadequate immune defenses

Wounds

- Acute pain related to trauma to nerve endings
- Impaired skin integrity related to penetration of skin
- Risk for contamination related to detrimental hospital or home environmental factors
- Risk for deficient fluid volume related to active loss from trauma
- Risk for infection related to inadequate primary defenses

Selected references

Ackley, B. J., Ladwig, G. B., & Makic, M. F. (2017). *Nursing diagnosis handbook: An evidence-based guide to planning care* (11th ed.). St. Louis, MO: Saunders.

Herdman, H., & Kamitsuru, S. (2014). *NANDA International, Inc. Nursing diagnoses: definitions & classification 2015–2017* (10th ed.). Wiley Blackwell. Retrieved on November 2016 from: http://iaud.ac.ir

Hinkle, J. L., & Cheever, K. H. (2014). *Brunner & Suddarth's textbook of medical-surgical nursing* (13th ed.). Philadelphia, PA: Wolters Kluwer.

Jalil, E. R. (2016). *NANDA nursing diagnosis list 2015–2017*. Retrieved on November 2016 from: http://health-conditions.com/nanda-nursing-diagnosis-list-2015-2017/

Lewis, S. L., Bucher, L., Heitkemper, M. M., & Harding, M. M. (2017). *Medical-surgical nursing: Assessment and management of clinical problems* (10th ed.). St. Louis, MO: Saunders.

NANDA International. *How do I write a diagnostic statement for risk, problem-focused and health promotion diagnoses?* Retrieved on December 2016 from: http://kb.nanda.org/article/AA-00492/36/English-/Frequently-Asked-Questions/Nursing-Diagnosis/Nursing-Diagnosis%3A-Learning-Using/How-do-I-write-a-diagnostic-statement-for-risk-problem-focused-and-health-promotion-diagnoses.html

Nettina, S. (2014). *Lippincott's manual of nursing practice* (10th ed.) New York: Lippincott Williams & Wilkins.

Chapter 9

Maternal-neonatal diagnoses

Just the facts

In this chapter, you'll learn:

♦ nursing diagnoses that correlate with common maternal-neonatal medical diagnoses.

A look at maternal-neonatal diagnoses

This chapter covers medical diagnoses that are applicable to pregnant patients and their neonates. Maternal-neonatal care can be complex because both the mother and neonate have many needs. The diagnoses listed here are just a sampling of the diagnoses that you might encounter on a maternity unit. Each entry provides a list of a few of the major nursing diagnoses and related factors to be considered after your assessment. Remember that the nursing diagnoses listed here represent the needs most commonly associated with the medical condition; your patient may have different needs.

Abortion

- Anxiety related to situational crisis
- Complicated grieving related to loss of pregnancy
- Moral distress related to decision and possible guilt
- Risk for complicated grieving related to pregnancy loss
- Risk for deficient fluid volume related to bleeding
- Risk for infection related to altered primary defenses
- Situational low self-esteem related to possible guilt
- Risk for decisional conflict
- Spiritual distress
- Acute pain

Abruptio placentae

- Acute pain related to separation of placenta
- Anxiety related to unknown outcome of pregnancy
- Deficient fluid volume related to bleeding
- Grieving related to potential loss of fetus

- Risk for decreased cardiac tissue perfusion (neonate) related to decreased cellular exchange
- Risk for development of coagulopathies (DIC [disseminated intravascular coagulation] and hyperfibrinogenemia)
- Risk for fetal hypoxia
- Risk for intrauterine infection
- Anemia related to blood loss
- Fear related to interventions and unknown outcomes
- Potential interrupted family process related to emergent status

Maternal-neonatal care must address the needs of both the mother and the neonate.

Acquired immunodeficiency syndrome

- Fear (parent) related to infant's future death as a result of human immunodeficiency virus (HIV) infection
- Risk for disturbed maternal-fetal dyad related to medication-related adverse effects
- Risk for infection related to:
  - immunosuppression
  - perinatal transmission of HIV
- Ineffective health maintenance related to lack of information and knowledge about HIV/AIDS
- Compromised family coping related to implications of positive HIV test in family member
- Grief related to recommendation to deter breast-feeding infant
- Risk for fatigue and activity intolerance
- Risk for ineffective coping related to progressive disease and complicated treatment regimen
- Situational or chronic low self-esteem related to chronic illness, isolation, and stigma of disease

Breast-feeding

- Deficient knowledge related to breast-feeding process, positioning, and techniques
- Ineffective breast-feeding related to newborn's inability to latch on
- Risk for infection related to mastitis
- Imbalanced nutrition: Less than body requirements related to:
  - lack of nutritional resources
  - poor intake
- Risk for impaired parenting related to unrealistic expectations of self and newborn regarding breast-feeding
- Anxiety related to lack of understanding about breast-feeding
- Risk for impaired parenting related to anxiety regarding breast-feeding outcomes
- Insufficient breast milk related to ineffective sucking
- Ineffective breast-feeding related to insufficient sucking
- Imbalanced nutrition less than body requirements

Cardiovascular disease in pregnancy

- Activity intolerance related to heart failure
- Decreased cardiac output related to heart decompensation and arrhythmias
- Risk for decreased cardiac tissue perfusion related to altered cardiovascular hemodynamics of pregnancy
- Risk for imbalanced fluid volume related to compromised regulatory mechanism
- Fear related to effects of maternal cardiac condition on fetal well-being and pregnancy outcome
- Risk for impaired gas exchange related to pulmonary edema secondary to cardiac decompensation
- Risk for fetal growth retardation/fetal injury

Cervical cerclage

- Acute pain related to surgical procedure
- Anxiety related to unknown outcome of pregnancy
- Deficient knowledge related to surgical procedure
- Fear related to possible loss of pregnancy
- Risk for infection related to surgical incision or procedure
- Anticipatory grieving related to potential loss of fetus, loss of normal pregnancy experience, premature delivery, and complications of premature newborn
- Powerlessness related to inability to control situation or prevent fetal loss

Cesarean birth

- Activity intolerance related to:
  - anesthetic administration
  - pain
  - surgical incision
- Acute pain related to surgical incision
- Ineffective coping related to:
  - fatigue
  - perceived loss of birthing experience
  - surgical intervention
- Readiness for enhanced parenting related to birth of healthy neonate
- Risk for deficient fluid volume related to bleeding associated with surgery
- Risk for infection related to:
  - bladder intubation
  - IV lines
  - repeated vaginal examination
  - sequela of anesthetic administration
  - surgical incision
- Fear related to unknown unpredictable maternal-fetal outcome
- Situational low self-esteem related to not having normal vaginal birth

Childbirth

- Acute pain related to physiological response to childbirth
- Anxiety related to hospitalization and birth process
- Deficient fluid volume related to altered intake during labor
- Deficient knowledge related to lack of information about birth process
- Impaired skin integrity related to episiotomy
- Impaired urinary elimination related to sensory impairment during labor
- Ineffective coping related to uncertainty about labor and birth
- Interrupted family processes related to:
  ○ impending birth
  ○ shift of roles to include new family member
- Readiness for enhanced breast-feeding related to basic breast-feeding knowledge
- Readiness for enhanced childbearing
- Readiness for enhanced parenting
- Risk for disturbed maternal-fetal dyad
- Risk for infection related to labor and birth
- Risk for injury related to labor

Many pregnant patients experience anxiety related to hospitalization and the birth process.

Cleft lip or palate

- Compromised family coping related to neonatal health problem
- Deficient knowledge (maternal) related to neonatal condition
- Imbalanced nutrition: Less than body requirements (neonate) related to altered nutritional intake
- Ineffective breast-feeding related to neonate's inability to latch onto nipple correctly due to structural anomaly of lip and palate
- Ineffective infant feeding pattern related to condition of lip and palate
- Risk for aspiration related to structural anomaly of lip and palate
- Interrupted family process related to stress and situational crisis and negative newborn outcome
- Deficient knowledge related to genetic testing procedures
- Decisional conflict related to lack of experience making decisions about treatment options
- Spiritual distress

Depression

- Risk for suicide risk or other directed violence
- Disturbed sleep pattern
- Risk due to impaired maternal/infant attachment
- Chronic and/or situational low self-esteem
- Risk for imbalanced nutrition: less than body requirements
- Powerlessness

- Anxiety
- Ineffective coping
- Interrupted family processes
- Risk for impaired parenting with other children

Diabetes mellitus and pregnancy

- Deficient fluid volume related to polyuria
- Deficient knowledge related to lack of information about disease
- Imbalanced nutrition: Less than body requirements related to inability to use glucose
- Imbalanced nutrition: More than body requirements related to altered carbohydrate metabolism
- Ineffective breathing pattern related to possible birth trauma in large-for-gestational-age neonate
- Ineffective breathing pattern related to uterine enlargement and excessive amniotic fluid
- Risk for disproportionate growth related to altered carbohydrate metabolism
- Risk for imbalanced nutrition: Less than body requirements (neonate) related to additional nutrients needed to maintain weight and prevent hypoglycemia
- Risk for impaired parenting related to high-risk status of neonate
- Risk for ineffective coping related to required change in lifestyle
- Risk for ineffective peripheral tissue perfusion related to reduced vascular flow
- Risk for infection related to disease process
- Risk for injury (fetal) related to dependence on maternal glycemic state
- Risk for injury related to birth trauma in large-for-gestational-age neonate
- Risk for unstable blood glucose level related to altered carbohydrate metabolism

Drug addiction and withdrawal

- Deficient knowledge (safe, healthy neonatal care, and development) related to emotional inadequacy and lack of exposure to information about infant care
- Imbalanced nutrition: Less than body requirements (neonate) related to:
  - poor or low intake because of lack of coordination in sucking or swallowing
  - vomiting
- Ineffective childbearing process related to deficient knowledge
- Ineffective coping (maternal) related to drug abuse or inability to care for the infant

- Ineffective infant feeding pattern related to delayed neurologic development
- Insufficient breast milk related to alcohol intake
- Risk for deficient fluid volume (neonate) related to diarrhea or vomiting
- Risk for impaired skin integrity (neonate) related to perianal irritation from diarrhea and rubbing against sheets because of hyperactivity
- Risk for ineffective childbearing process related to deficient knowledge
- Risk for injury (neonate) related to withdrawal from drug exposure
- Risk for ineffective breathing pattern (newborn) related to meconium aspiration syndrome due to fetal stress and hypoxia
- Impaired parenting related to hyperirritable behavior of the infant and lack of knowledge of infant care
- Risk for respiratory distress syndrome
- Risk for sudden infant death syndrome (SIDS)
- Risk for premature pregnancy outcome
- Risk for intrauterine growth retardation

Ectopic pregnancy

- Acute pain related to disruption of pelvic tissue
- Anxiety related to situational crisis
- Deficient fluid volume related to bleeding
- Fear related to loss of pregnancy and threat to future fertility
- Risk for imbalanced fluid volume related to concealed hemorrhage and blood loss
- Risk for infection related to the trauma of tubal rupture and peritoneal inflammation
- Situational low self-esteem related to loss of perceived pregnancy
- Risk for Rh sensitization
- Anticipatory grieving related to loss of pregnancy and possible loss of fertility

Fetal alcohol syndrome

- Deficient knowledge (parental) related to lack of information about infant care
- Delayed growth and development (neonate) related to neurologic and mental deficiency
- Dysfunctional family processes: Alcoholism related to abuse of alcohol
- Imbalanced nutrition: Less than body requirements (neonate) related to:
  - lack of nutritional resources
  - poor intake

- Risk for disproportionate growth related to imbalanced nutrition and poor intake
- Risk for impaired parenting related to:
  - lifestyle associated with alcohol abuse
  - unrealistic expectations of self and neonate
- Risk for neonatal jaundice related to difficulty in making the transition to extrauterine life

Fetal alcohol syndrome can cause delays in growth and development.

Fetal/newborn death

- Dysfunctional grieving
- Powerlessness
- Situational low self-esteem
- Anxiety
- Risk for interrupted family processes
- Spiritual distress
- Risk for impaired parenting with other children
- Interrupted family processes
- Ineffective coping
- Anticipatory grieving
- Risk for imbalanced nutrition: less than body requirements

Hemorrhage

- Risk for deficient fluid volume related to active blood loss
- Decreased tissue perfusion related to blood loss
- Acute pain related to episiotomy/hematoma/laceration
- Risk for impaired parenting due to:
  - fear related to unknown maternal-fetal outcome
  - anxiety related to blood loss
- Impaired/ineffective coping related to situational crisis
- Risk for impaired parenting related to maternal blood loss
- Risk for fetal injury related to uteroplacental insufficiency
- Risk for complication of postpartum hematoma

Hydrocephalus

- Anxiety (parent) related to lack of understanding about the child's condition and treatment
- Compromised family coping related to illness of neonate
- Deficient knowledge (maternal) related to health care needs of child with hydrocephalus
- Delayed growth and development related to disease
- Imbalanced nutrition: Less than body requirements related to feeding difficulties
- Interrupted family processes (maternal) related to impact on family of neonate's disorder
- Risk for deficient fluid volume related to altered nutritional status

- Risk for impaired skin integrity related to extra weight and immobility of child's head
- Risk for ineffective cerebral tissue perfusion related to increased intracranial pressure
- Risk for infection related to surgical placement of shunt
- Risk for injury related to onset of seizures

Hyperemesis gravidarum

- Deficient fluid volume related to protracted emesis
- Fear related to hospitalization and pregnancy outcome
- Imbalanced nutrition: Less than body requirements related to nausea and vomiting and insufficient food intake
- Nausea due to hormonal changes related to pregnancy
- Impaired home maintenance

Hypertension of pregnancy

- Activity intolerance related to activity restrictions
- Deficient fluid volume related to compromised regulatory mechanisms
- Deficient knowledge (signs and symptoms of increased blood pressure) related to lack of exposure to information
- Excess fluid volume related to compromised regulatory mechanisms
- Fear related to unknown outcome of pregnancy
- Risk for ineffective cerebral tissue perfusion related to compromised regulatory mechanisms
- Risk for injury (fetal) related to impaired maternal-placental perfusion
- Urinary retention related to compromised regulatory mechanisms
- Risk for hemorrhage secondary to placental separation, HELLP syndrome, or DIC

Infection

- Risk for infection related to labor and birth process
- Pain related to presence of infectious site
- Risk for infection related to secondary infection of mastitis
- Risk for infection related to urinary stasis and over distention of bladder
- Risk for delayed parent-infant attachment secondary to malaise, other symptoms of infection, and separation of mother and newborn
- Risk for injury related to spread of infection
- Risk of infection related to episiotomy and surgical procedures

Mastitis

- Acute pain secondary to milk stasis
- Risk of interrupted breast-feeding related to knowledge deficiency
- Risk for infection related to milk stasis
- Ineffective breast-feeding related to pain secondary to development of mastitis
- Risk for trauma related to knowledge deficient and lack of information related to appropriate breast-feeding process
- Anxiety relayed interruption in breast-feeding process
- Ineffective coping related to inability to breast-feed secondary to mastitis
- Risk for disturbance in parenting related to development of breast-feeding process
- Interrupted breast-feeding

Meconium aspiration syndrome

- Disabled family coping related to anxiety and guilt
- Impaired gas exchange related to:
  - impaired alveoli capillary changes
  - ventilation-perfusion imbalance
- Impaired spontaneous ventilation related to respiratory muscle fatigue
- Ineffective breathing pattern related to meconium aspiration
- Interrupted breast-feeding related to need for ventilatory support
- Risk for aspiration related to presence of meconium
- Risk for injury related to meconium aspiration
- Impaired parent-infant attachment
- Imbalanced nutrition: Less than body requirements related to respiratory distress and increased energy requirements
- Interrupted family process related to threatening illness in term newborn

Multiple gestation

- Anxiety related to unknown outcome of pregnancy
- Deficient knowledge related to unknown outcome of pregnancy
- Impaired parenting related to demands of caring for multiple neonates
- Ineffective coping related to dramatic increase in family size
- Risk for impaired parenting related to anxiety regarding caring for multiple neonates
- Risk for injury related to:
  - physiological demands of multifetal pregnancy (maternal and fetal)
  - preterm labor and birth (maternal and fetal)

- Stress urinary incontinence related to increased weight of gravid uterus on bladder
- Risk for hydramnios related to increase renal perfusion from cross-vessel anastomosis of monozygotic twins
- Discomfort related to shortness of breath, dyspnea on exertion, backache, and/or pedal edema
- Risk for activity intolerance related to increased energy requirements, fatigue, and sleep disturbance
- Imbalanced nutrition: Less than body requirement related to increased metabolic needs of mother and fetuses, nausea, and vomiting
- Constipation related to compression of bowel by enlarged uterus and multiple fetuses

A dramatic increase in family size can lead to ineffective coping. Sure, these two can be a handful, but imagine trying to juggle quadruplets.

Myelomeningocele

- Delayed growth and development related to spinal cord dysfunction
- Impaired skin integrity related to presence of myelomeningocele and surgical procedure
- Impaired urinary elimination related to injury of spinal nerves
- Imbalanced nutrition: Less than body requirements related to surgery
- Risk for impaired parenting related to maternal separation from the neonate at birth
- Interrupted family processes related to disruption of usual family functions, stress, situational crisis, and unpredictable or negative outcomes
- Grief related to situational crisis and threat to newborn
- Anxiety related to situational crisis, interventions, procedures, and newborn treatments
- Spiritual distress related to infant anomaly

Necrotizing enterocolitis

- Diarrhea related to inflammation
- Ineffective infant feeding pattern related to nothing-by-mouth status
- Interrupted family processes related to shift in health status of family member

Neural tube defects

- Decisional conflict (possible abortion) related to genetic defect
- Interrupted family processes related to change in health status of family member

- Spiritual distress related to chronic illness
- Anxiety related to situational crisis
- Grief related to situational crisis and threat to pregnancy

Placenta previa

- Anxiety related to unknown hospital procedures
- Deficient fluid volume related to active loss, bleeding
- Fear related to unknown maternal and fetal outcome
- Risk for injury (fetal) related to uteroplacental insufficiency
- Impaired gas exchange (fetus) related to decreased blood volume and maternal hypotension
- Risk for intrauterine infection

Premature rupture of membranes

- Anxiety related to situational crisis
- Risk for infection related to lack of primary defenses
- Risk for umbilical cord prolapse
- Risk for impaired gas exchange (fetus) related to compression of the umbilical cord secondary to prolapse of the cord
- Ineffective coping related to unknown outcome of the pregnancy

Preterm labor

- Anxiety related to unknown outcome of pregnancy
- Deficient knowledge related to procedures
- Impaired parenting related to inadequate attachment to high-risk neonate
- Ineffective breast-feeding related to prematurity of neonate and insufficient sucking
- Insufficient breast milk related to ineffective sucking
- Risk for disturbed maternal-fetal dyad related to separation from neonate at birth
- Risk for neonatal jaundice related to prematurity
- Risk for infection related to possible premature rupture of membranes
- Situational low self-esteem related to guilt about preterm labor

Respiratory distress syndrome

- Impaired gas exchange related to:
  - dysfunctional alveolar ventilation
  - dysfunctional lung perfusion
  - reduced lung volume and compliance
- Ineffective airway clearance related to immature respiratory functioning

- Ineffective breathing pattern related to impaired adjustment to extrauterine environment
- Decreased cardiac output related to pulmonary disease
- Imbalanced nutrition: Less than body requirements related to:
  - decreased gastric motility
  - inability to digest feedings
  - withholding of food and water
- Ineffective thermoregulation related to immaturity
- Risk for deficient fluid volume related to active fluid losses
- Risk for injury related to medical therapy and treatments
- Disabled family coping related to anxiety, guilt, and separation from the infant as a result of situational crisis

Uterine rupture

- Risk for impaired gas exchange (fetus) related to decreased blood flow secondary to uterine rupture
- Risk for impaired gas exchange in mother related to decrease blood flow secondary to uterine rupture
- Fear related to unknown outcome
- Anxiety related to emergent procedures and unknown outcome
- Impaired/ineffective coping due to emergent situation
- Acute abdominal pain secondary to uterine rupture
- Risk for complications related to hypovolemia and decreased cardiac output secondary to uterine rupture
- Risk for changes in mental status related to decreased oxygenation and blood flow to the brain secondary to uterine rupture
- Risk for delayed and ineffective maternal/newborn attachment
- Risk for impaired parenting related to secondary uterine rupture
- Ineffective or delayed breast-feeding related to maternal uterine rupture
- Ineffective coping related to perceived loss of birthing experience
- Ineffective coping related to surgical intervention
- Risk for deficient fluid volume related to blood loss
- Interruption in family processes related to shift in roles to include new family member
- Compromised family coping related to maternal bleeding
- Deficient knowledge related to unknown outcome
- Ineffective tissue perfusion

Selected references

Carpenito, L. H. (2017). *Nursing diagnosis application to clinical practice* (15th ed.). Philadelphia, PA: Wolters Kluwer.

Green, C. J., & Wilkinson, J. M. (2004). *Maternal newborn nursing care plans*. St. Louis, MO: Mosby. Reprinted from Publication with permission from Elsevier, pp.119–128, 186–197, 211–242, 254–288, 591–593, 661–662.

Herdman, T. H., & Kamitsuru, S. (Eds.). (2014). *Nanda international nursing diagnosis: Definitions and classifications 2015–2017*. Oxford, UK: Wiley Blackwell.

Ladewig, P. A., London, M. L., & Davidson, M. R. (2014). *Contemporary maternal-child newborn nursing care* (8th ed.). Boston, MA: Pearson.

Lowdermilk, D. L., Perry, S. E., Cashion, K., Alden, K. R., & Olshansky, E. F. (2016). *Maternity and women's health care* (11th ed.). Philadelphia, PA: Elsevier.

Chapter 10

Pediatric diagnoses

Just the facts

In this chapter, you'll learn:

♦ nursing diagnoses that correlate with common pediatric medical diagnoses.

A look at pediatric diagnoses

This chapter covers medical diagnoses that are common in pediatric patients. Remember that pediatric patients can have the same medical and nursing diagnoses as an adult; however, the care provided for these patients may be different. Each entry provides a list of a few of the major nursing diagnoses and related factors to be considered after your assessment. Remember that the nursing diagnoses listed here represent the needs most commonly associated with the medical condition in pediatric patients; your pediatric patient may have different needs.

> Although pediatric patients can have the same diagnoses as adults, the care provided may be different.

Acne vulgaris

- Deficient knowledge (care of skin) related to lack of exposure to information
- Situational low self-esteem related to face lesions
- Social isolation related to alteration in physical appearance
- Risk for depression related to poor body image

Anorexia nervosa

- Deficient fluid volume related to active loss
- Disturbed body image related to psychological effects of the disorder
- Imbalanced nutrition: Less than body requirements related to fear of obesity
- Impaired social interaction related to low self-esteem
- Interrupted family processes related to illness of family member
- Social isolation related to eating habits

- Readiness for enhanced nutrition related to treatment for anorexia nervosa
- Risk for depression related to psychological effects of the disorder
- Risk for suicide related to psychological effects of disorder
- Risk for self-mutilation related to disturbed eating habits

Aplastic and hypoplastic anemias

- Activity intolerance related to imbalance between oxygen supply and demand
- Fatigue related to disease process
- Ineffective breathing pattern related to weakness and fatigue
- Ineffective family coping related to altered health status of family member
- Risk for infection related to destruction of stem cells in bone marrow
- Complicated grieving related to chronic illness
- Interrupted breast-feeding due to infant's weakness and breathing difficulty

Arm and leg fractures

- Bathing, dressing, feeding self-care deficit related to immobility of affected limb
- Impaired walking related to cast or splints
- Risk for injury related to inability to use body part

Asthma

- Activity intolerance related to imbalance between oxygen supply and demand
- Anxiety related to threat to health status
- Deficient knowledge (home care procedures) related to new diagnosis
- Deficient knowledge (treatment regimen) related to complexity of therapeutic regimen
- Fatigue related to hypoxia
- Impaired gas exchange related to bronchial constriction
- Ineffective airway clearance related to constriction
- Readiness for enhanced self-health management related to perceived benefits
- Risk for allergy response to iodinized contrast media related to diagnostic procedure
- Risk for deficient fluid volume related to loss of fluid from the respiratory tract

Attention deficit hyperactivity disorder

- Impaired social interaction related to hyperactivity
- Interrupted family processes related to shift in health status of family member

- Risk for delayed development related to brain disorder
- Moderate to severe anxiety related to hyperactivity
- Readiness for enhanced communication related to treatment for ADHD
- Readiness for enhanced family coping related to treatment for ADHD

Autism spectrum disorder

- Impaired social interaction related to brain disorder
- Impaired verbal communication related to stimulus confusion
- Risk for impaired parenting related to 24-hour demands of child with special needs
- Risk for other-directed or self-directed violence related to impaired capacity to identify and express feelings
- Readiness for enhanced family processes related to child's needs
- Stress overload related to child's needs

Biliary atresia

- Deficient fluid volume related to poor absorption of nutrients
- Deficient knowledge (home care procedures) related to new diagnosis
- Risk for delayed development related to chronic illness
- Risk for disproportionate growth related to chronic illness
- Risk for electrolyte imbalance due to liver dysfunction
- Jaundice related to liver dysfunction
- Impaired liver function due to biliary atresia
- Readiness for enhanced nutrition related to treatment for biliary atresia

Bronchiolitis

- Anxiety (child and parent) related to lack of knowledge about condition
- Deficient knowledge (home care procedures) related to new diagnosis
- Fatigue related to respiratory distress
- Hyperthermia related to infection
- Imbalanced nutrition: Less than body requirements related to:
  - inability to take oral feeding
  - increased metabolic needs
- Impaired gas exchange related to bronchiolar edema and increased mucus production
- Risk for deficient fluid volume related to increased water loss through exhalation and decreased fluid intake
- Social isolation related to isolation precautions
- Interrupted breast-feeding related to infant's breathing difficulty

Bronchopulmonary dysplasia

- Anxiety (parent) related to fear and lack of knowledge about the child's illness
- Imbalanced nutrition: Less than body requirements related to increased metabolic rate and high calorie demands
- Impaired gas exchange related to atelectasis
- Risk for delayed development related to chronic illness, prematurity, or prolonged hospitalization
- Risk for disproportionate growth related to chronic illness, prematurity, or prolonged hospitalization
- Risk for impaired parenting related to chronic illness
- Risk for impaired skin integrity related to irritation from nasogastric tube feedings
- Interrupted breast-feeding due to infant's breathing difficulty

Bulimia nervosa

- Constipation related to poor eating habits and insufficient fluid intake
- Deficient fluid volume related to active loss
- Disturbed body image related to illness
- Disturbed personal identity related to body weight
- Imbalanced nutrition: Less than body requirements related to binge-purge behavior
- Readiness for enhanced nutrition related to treatment for bulimia nervosa
- Risk for self-mutilation related to disturbed eating habits
- Social isolation related to eating disorder

Keep in mind that many pediatric conditions cause anxiety in parents and other family members or caregivers.

Cerebral palsy

- Bathing self-care deficit related to involuntary movements and impaired muscle function
- Caregiver role strain related to complex needs of care recipient
- Impaired physical mobility related to impaired muscle function
- Impaired swallowing related to impaired muscle function
- Risk for aspiration related to impaired motor activity
- Risk for delayed development related to neuromuscular impairment
- Risk for disproportionate growth related to neuromuscular impairment
- Risk for nutrition, less than body requirements due to child's neuromuscular impairment
- Readiness for enhanced family processes related to treatment for child's disorder
- Caregiver fatigue related to child's complex needs

- Risk for fluid volume deficit related to child's impaired muscle function
- Risk for impaired home maintenance due to child's care needs
- Social isolation related to child's impairments and complex needs

Child abuse

- Impaired parenting related to the abusive parent's inability to attach to or bond with the child
- Ineffective family coping related to personal issues that contribute to child abuse
- Risk for delayed development related to inadequate caregiving
- Risk for disproportionate growth related to inadequate caregiving
- Risk for other-directed violence (abusive family member) related to maladaptive behavior
- Nutrition, risk for less than body requirements related to inadequate caregiving
- Risk for depression and suicide related to child despair
- Social isolation related to inadequate caregiving

Cleft lip and cleft palate

- Disabled family coping related to the stress of hospitalization (preoperative)
- Imbalanced nutrition: Less than body requirements related to impaired feeding (preoperative)
- Impaired skin integrity related to surgical incision
- Ineffective infant feeding pattern related to deformity
- Risk for aspiration related to ineffective feeding
- Risk for perioperative positioning injury related to surgical repair
- Interrupted breast-feeding due to child's inability to suck effectively
- Impaired dentition due to child's malformation of mouth
- Risk for situational low self-esteem related to congenital anomalies

Clubfoot

- Compromised family coping related to situational crisis
- Deficient knowledge (treatment protocols) related to lack of exposure to information
- Impaired physical mobility related to casting or splinting
- Risk for delayed development related to impaired early ambulation
- Risk for disproportionate growth related to impaired early ambulation
- Risk for impaired skin integrity related to casting or splinting
- Risk for injury related to failure to provide appropriate care, leading to complications
- Risk for peripheral neurovascular dysfunction related to casting of limb

Complement deficiency
- Deficient knowledge (treatment options) related to lack of exposure to information
- Disabled family coping related to change in health status of family member
- Risk for infection related to increased susceptibility to infection

Congenital heart defect
- Anxiety (child) related to:
  - immobility
  - intensive care unit environment
  - parental anxiety
  - separation from parents
  - surgery
- Anxiety (parent) related to child's congenital heart defect
- Decreased cardiac output related to congenital cardiac anomalies and surgical procedures
- Deficient knowledge (preoperative and postoperative care) related to impending surgery
- Risk for adverse reaction to iodinated contrast media related to diagnostic procedure
- Risk for delayed development related to congenital heart defect
- Risk for disproportionate growth related to congenital heart defect
- Risk for infection related to immobility and numerous incisions
- Risk for injury related to:
  - blood loss
  - electric current
  - positioning
  - surgical procedure

Congenital hip dysplasia
- Constipation related to immobility and opiate-based treatment
- Impaired comfort related to hip joint abnormality
- Risk for disproportionate growth related to hip joint abnormality
- Knowledge deficit related to traction or spica cast
- Impaired mobility due to hip joint abnormality
- Deficient diversional activity related to immobility secondary to traction or spica cast
- Risk for impaired skin integrity related to:
  - immobility
  - spica cast
  - traction
- Risk for infection related to break in skin integrity secondary to traction (if pins are used)
- Risk for injury related to possible mechanical malfunctioning of traction or circulatory compromise

Croup

- Anxiety related to hospitalization and respiratory distress
- Impaired gas exchange related to bronchial secretion accumulation and bronchospasm
- Ineffective airway clearance related to laryngeal obstruction
- Ineffective breathing pattern related to upper airway edema and thickened secretions
- Risk for deficient fluid volume related to decreased oral intake
- Risk for infection related to break in primary defenses
- Infection related to viral illness

Cystic fibrosis

- Anxiety (child) related to respiratory distress and hospitalization
- Anxiety (parent) related to lack of knowledge about the child's condition
- Delayed growth and development related to autosomal recessive genetic inheritance
- Fear related to inability to breath
- Impaired gas exchange related to increased mucus production by exocrine glands
- Deficient knowledge (home care procedures) related to complex disorder
- Deficient knowledge related to genetic basis for illness
- Imbalanced nutrition: Less than body requirements related to reduced absorption of nutrients
- Impaired gas exchange related to increased mucus production
- Parental role conflict related to child's hospitalization
- Risk for delayed development related to chronic illness
- Risk for disproportionate growth related to chronic illness
- Risk for infection related to increased mucus production

Down syndrome

- Risk for impaired cardiovascular function related to congenital disorder
- Readiness for enhanced communication related to family caregiving
- Readiness for enhanced family and community coping related to needs of child
- Delayed growth and development related to chromosomal abnormality (translocation or trisomy 21)
- Interrupted family processes related to child's developmental disability
- Knowledge deficit related to family genetic risk
- Readiness for enhanced parenting related to child's needs
- Readiness for enhanced relationship related to child's needs
- Risk for impaired resilience due to chronic complex needs of child

- Risk for delayed development related to chromosomal abnormality
- Social isolation related to child's congenital disorder and complex needs
- Chronic sorrow related to child's congenital disorder and complex needs

Epiglottitis

- Anxiety (parent) related to lack of knowledge concerning the child's condition
- Infection due to bacterial illness
- Fear, air hunger, and drooling due to inflamed and edematous airway
- Anxiety and fear (child) related to respiratory distress and hospitalization
- Disabled family coping related to anxiety and fear
- Hyperthermia related to infection
- Impaired swallowing related to inflammation and edema
- Ineffective airway clearance related to inflammation and edema
- Ineffective breathing pattern related to upper airway edema
- Risk for aspiration related to excessive production of oral secretions
- Risk for deficient fluid volume related to decreased intake

Esophagitis, corrosive

- Impaired parenting related to:
  - deficient knowledge about injury protection
  - poor home environment
  - presence of stress
- Ineffective feeding pattern of child or infant related to esophageal disorder
- Risk for disproportionate growth related to esophageal disorder
- Readiness for enhanced knowledge related to parenting and care of child
- Risk for poisoning related to presence of poison within reach of child
- Nutrition, less than body requirements related to esophageal disorder

Fracture

- Acute pain related to muscle spasm, swelling, or bleeding
- Constipation related to immobility and opiate-based treatment
- Feeding self-care deficit related to limb cast and immobility
- Impaired gas exchange related to complications secondary to the fracture and immobility

- Ineffective peripheral tissue perfusion related to:
  - bleeding
  - cast
  - swelling
  - traction
- Risk for activity intolerance related to immobility from cast or traction
- Risk for impaired skin integrity related to immobility from cast or traction
- Toileting self-care deficit related to limb cast and immobility

Fragile X syndrome

- Impaired verbal communication related to intellectual disability
- Interrupted family processes related to shift in health status of family member
- Readiness for enhanced family and community coping related to child's complex needs
- Delayed growth and development related to X-linked dominant gene inheritance
- Impaired verbal communication related to developmental delay
- Interrupted family processes related to developmental disability
- Readiness for enhanced parenting related to child's complex needs
- Readiness for enhanced relationship related to child caregiving
- Risk for impaired resilience related to child's complex needs
- Risk for caregiver role strain related to complex care needs of care recipient
- Social isolation related to child's complex needs
- Chronic sorrow related to child's complex health problems and needs

Glycogen storage disease

- Anxiety (parent) related to lack of knowledge concerning the child's condition
- Readiness for enhanced nutrition related to readiness to manage disease through diet
- Risk for delayed development related to chronic illness
- Risk for disproportionate growth related to chronic illness
- Readiness for enhanced communication related to chronic illness of child
- Readiness for enhanced family and community coping due to child's needs
- Delayed growth and development related to recessive genetic inheritance
- Impaired verbal communication related to developmental delay
- Interrupted family processes related to developmental disability
- Deficient knowledge related to family genetic risk

- Readiness for enhanced parenting related to caregiving of child
- Readiness for enhanced nutrition related to management of disease through diet
- Risk for impaired resilience related to child's complex needs
- Risk for caregiver role strain related to complex care needs of care recipient
- Social isolation due to child's complex needs
- Chronic sorrow related to child's complex needs

Haemophilus influenzae infection

- Deficient fluid volume related to active loss
- Hyperthermia related to infection
- Impaired gas exchange related to ventilation-perfusion imbalance
- Infection due to bacterial illness
- Deficient family and community knowledge of immunizations, *Haemophilus influenzae* B vaccine

Head injury/concussion

- Acute pain related to head injury
- Anxiety (child and parent) related to traumatic head injury
- Decreased intracranial adaptive capacity related to cerebral edema
- Deficient knowledge (home care procedures) related to new diagnosis
- Deficient knowledge related to concussion management
- Ineffective breathing pattern (with potential for respiratory failure) related to increased intracranial pressure (ICP)
- Risk for deficient fluid volume related to nausea and vomiting
- Risk for impaired skin integrity related to physical immobility
- Risk for infection related to injury
- Risk for injury related to altered level of consciousness secondary to head injury or increased ICP (or both)
- Risk for delayed development related to brain injury
- Risk for injury secondary to seizures

Traumatic head injury can cause anxiety for both the child and the parent. What if my head never stops spinning?

Hemophilia

- Acute pain related to bleeding and swelling
- Chronic low self-esteem related to chronic illness and hospitalization
- Compromised family coping related to repeated hospitalization and the child's chronic illness
- Impaired physical mobility related to decreased range of motion secondary to bleeding and swelling
- Risk for bleeding related to insufficient functioning of clotting cascade

- Risk for injury (hemorrhage) related to disease
- Anxiety related to possibility of hemorrhage and death
- Delayed growth and development related to X-linked recessive genetic inheritance
- Impaired health management related to low hemoglobin and hematocrit
- Deficient knowledge related to family genetic risk

Hirschsprung's disease

- Anxiety (parent) related to lack of knowledge about the disease and prescribed treatment
- Constipation related to neuromuscular impairment of colon
- Disturbed body image related to colostomy or ileostomy
- Impaired skin integrity related to exposure to stools secondary to colostomy or ileostomy
- Risk for adverse reaction to iodinated contrast media related to diagnostic procedure
- Risk for deficient fluid volume related to:
  - decreased intake
  - increased absorptive surface of distended bowel
  - nausea and vomiting
- Risk for infection of incision related to contamination from stools
- Delayed growth and development related to complex genetic inheritance pattern
- Knowledge, deficient related to family genetic risk

Hypopituitarism

- Anxiety related to treatment regimen
- Risk for delayed development related to deficiency of anterior pituitary hormones
- Risk for disproportionate growth related to deficiency of anterior pituitary hormones
- Risk for injury related to lack of proper medication administration

Hypospadias and epispadias

- Acute pain related to surgery
- Anxiety (child and parent) related to surgical procedure (urethroplasty)
- Impaired tissue integrity related to surgical repair
- Risk for infection (urinary tract) related to placement of indwelling catheter
- Risk for injury related to dislodged urinary catheter or urinary catheter removal
- Risk for low situational self-esteem related to congenital anomaly

Impetigo

- Deficient knowledge (parent, treatment and prevention of recurrence of infection) related to new diagnosis
- Impaired skin integrity related to skin infection
- Risk for infection related to inadequate immune defenses

Intraventricular hemorrhage related to prematurity

- Deficient knowledge (infant's condition and potential for home care) related to the new injury
- Risk for injury related to fragility of the capillary beds in the cerebrum
- See head injury

Intussusception

- Acute pain related to bowel strangulation
- Anxiety (parent) related to infant's pain and surgery
- Nausea and vomiting due to intestinal disorder
- Risk for adverse reaction to iodinated contrast media related to diagnostic procedure
- Risk for infection related to gangrenous bowel
- Risk for delayed surgical recovery

Juvenile rheumatoid arthritis

- Activity intolerance related to severe joint pain and edema
- Chronic pain related to joint inflammation
- Disturbed body image related to the effects of the chronic illness and the disabling nature of the disease
- Dressing self-care deficit related to severe joint pain and edema
- Impaired physical mobility related to joint inflammation
- Impaired skin integrity related to immobility
- Risk for imbalanced body temperature related to disease process
- Readiness for enhanced coping related to treatment of disorder
- Risk for chronic low self-esteem related to disorder
- Impaired walking due to joint inflammation and edema

Kyphosis/kyphoscoliosis

- Disturbed body image related to altered physical appearance
- Readiness for enhanced management of therapeutic regimen related to readiness to follow treatment regimen
- Risk for situational low self-esteem related to altered physical appearance

Leukemia, acute

- Delayed growth and development related to treatment regimen
- Risk for infection related to immunosuppression

- Fatigue related to pancytopenia
- Hopelessness related to illness
- Impaired oral mucous membrane related to chemotherapy adverse effects
- Ineffective protection related to immunosuppression
- Risk for imbalanced body temperature related to infection
- Compromised family coping due to child's disorder
- Readiness for enhanced family coping related to altered health status of family member
- Interrupted family processes related to child's disorder
- Anxiety-related potential fatality of illness
- Risk for loneliness related to child's disorder

Mononucleosis

- Fatigue related to weakness
- Interrupted family processes related to family member becoming temporary full-time caregiver
- Risk for imbalanced body temperature related to infection
- Ineffective thermoregulation due to infection

Muscular dystrophy

- Caregiver role strain related to increased care needs
- Dressing self-care deficit related to muscle weakness and disability
- Impaired physical mobility related to muscle weakness
- Ineffective health maintenance related to inability to care for self
- Hopelessness related to prognosis of muscular dystrophy
- Compromised family coping related to degenerative neurologic disease
- Delayed development related to degenerative genetic disease
- Deficient knowledge related to family genetic risk
- Chronic sorrow related to degenerative changes of disease
- Impaired walking due to neurological degenerative disease

Myringotomy

- Anxiety (child and parent) related to the surgical procedure and perioperative events
- Deficient knowledge (home care procedures) related to new treatment
- Risk for injury (hemorrhage) related to surgery
- Risk for infection related to surgical procedure of middle ear

Osteomyelitis

- Chronic pain related to inflammation and infection
- Compromised family coping related to prolonged hospitalization
- Imbalanced nutrition: Less than body requirements related to increased metabolic needs for wound healing

- Impaired physical mobility related to infection
- Impaired skin integrity related to infection
- Risk for infection related to wound contamination
- Impaired walking due to bone infection of limb

Otitis media

- Acute pain related to inflammation of the middle ear
- Disturbed sensory perception (auditory) related to complications of otitis media
- Infection related to viral or bacterial illness

Pediculosis

- Impaired skin integrity related to itching and redness
- Situational low self-esteem related to lice
- Social isolation related to feelings of embarrassment due to diagnosis
- Deficient knowledge related to life cycle of lice
- Ineffective family and community coping due to contagion of disease
- Readiness for enhanced family and community coping related to treatment of disease

Some children with otitis media experience acute pain related to inflammation.

Phenylketonuria

- Disturbed thought processes related to intellectual disability
- Impaired skin integrity related to dry skin lesions
- Risk for delayed development related to accumulation of phenyl-alanine in blood
- Interrupted breast-feeding of infant due to genetic disorder
- Delayed development related to autosomal recessive genetic inheritance
- Deficient knowledge related to family genetic risk

Pyloric stenosis

- Acute pain related to surgical incision
- Anxiety (parent) related to lack of understanding about the disease, diagnostic studies, and treatment
- Risk for deficient fluid volume related to dehydration or shock (or both)
- Imbalanced nutrition: Less than body requirements related to frequent projectile vomiting
- Risk for infection related to surgery
- Deficient knowledge related to family genetic risk
- Nausea and vomiting related to hypertrophy of pyloric sphincter and valve occlusion

Respiratory syncytial virus infection

- Imbalanced nutrition: Less than body requirements related to inability to ingest foods
- Ineffective breathing pattern related to decreased energy
- Risk for deficient fluid volume related to active loss and inflamed mucous membranes of the throat

Rheumatic fever and rheumatic heart disease

- Acute pain related to joint pain
- Decreased cardiac output related to carditis
- Hyperthermia related to infection
- Impaired gas exchange related to diminished pumping action of heart

Roseola infantum

- Deficient knowledge (child's care needs and prognosis) related to infection
- Hyperthermia related to viral infection
- Impaired skin integrity related to rash

Rubella

- Ineffective coping of family and community related to immunizations and disease prevention
- Deficient knowledge related to infection (child's care needs and prognosis)
- Deficient knowledge of family and community related to immunizations and disease prevention
- Hyperthermia related to infection
- Risk for fetal injury
- Impaired skin integrity related to rash
- Risk for disturbed maternal-fetal dyad
- Hyperthermia related to infection
- Impaired skin integrity related to rash

Rubeola

- Fatigue related to infection
- Hyperthermia related to infection
- Impaired skin integrity related to pruritic rash
- Ineffective coping of family and community related to immunizations and disease prevention
- Deficient knowledge related to infection (child's care needs and prognosis)
- Deficient knowledge of family and community related to immunizations and disease

Scoliosis

- Acute pain related to curvature of spine
- Disturbed body image related to altered body shape
- Risk for injury during perioperative period related to surgery
- Pain related to surgery
- Risk for impaired skin integrity related to brace
- Risk for situational low self-esteem related to altered physical appearance

Sickle cell anemia

- Acute pain related to vascular occlusion and tissue hypoxia
- Deficient fluid volume related to decreased fluid intake and the kidneys' inability to concentrate urine
- Deficient knowledge related to sickle cell crisis prevention
- Impaired gas exchange related to decreased oxygen-carrying capacity of blood
- Ineffective peripheral tissue perfusion related to blood vessel obstruction secondary to sickling of red blood cells
- Delayed growth and development related to genetic disorder
- Risk for injury due to vasoocclusive crisis in vital organs and extremities
- Acute pain due to sickle cell vasoocclusive crises
- Chronic pain due to sickle cell vasoocclusive crises

Spinal cord defects

- Deficient knowledge (spinal cord defects) related to lack of exposure to information
- Disabled family coping related to increased caregiving demands on family with minimal social support
- Risk for delayed development related to spinal cord defect
- Risk for disproportionate growth related to spinal cord defect
- Risk for overflow urinary incontinence due to spinal cord defect
- Risk for infection related to immobility
- Risk for injury related to immobility

Tay-Sachs disease

- Disabled family coping related to family member with unexpressed feelings of anxiety
- Grieving related to death of child
- Risk for delayed development related to muscle weakness
- Risk for disproportionate growth related to muscle weakness
- Deficient knowledge related to autosomal recessive genetic inheritance
- Readiness for enhanced family coping related to child's disorder

Tonsillitis

- Acute pain related to throat swelling
- Hyperthermia related to infection
- Impaired swallowing related to swelling

Tracheoesophageal fistula

- Anxiety (parent) related to lack of knowledge about the disorder, diagnostic testing, and treatment
- Ineffective airway clearance related to aspiration of secretions or feedings or both
- Ineffective breathing pattern related to choking, coughing, and cyanosis during feeding
- Risk for adverse reaction to iodinated contrast media related to diagnostic procedure
- Risk for delayed development related to hospitalization and deprivation of normal parent-infant interactions and environmental stimulation
- Risk for disproportionate growth related to hospitalization and deprivation of normal parent-infant interactions and environmental stimulation
- Interrupted breast-feeding due to infant's tracheoesophageal disorder

Tympanoplasty

- Anxiety (child and parent) related to surgical procedure and perioperative events
- Risk for injury (hemorrhage) related to surgery
- Risk for infection related to surgery

Varicella zoster

- Acute pain related to rash
- Impaired skin integrity related to pruritic rash
- Interrupted family processes related to family member having to stay home from work to care for child
- Ineffective coping of family and community related to immunizations and disease prevention
- Deficient knowledge of family and community related to immunizations and disease prevention
- Hyperthermia related to infection

Tonsillitis can cause pain and difficulty swallowing. Luckily, ice cream slides right down!

Selected references

Ackley, B., & Ladwig, G. (2014). *Nursing diagnosis handbook: An evidenced-based guide to planning care* (10th ed.). St. Louis, MO: Elsevier-Mosby.

Doenges, M. E., Moorhouse, M. F., & Murr, A. C. (2016). *Nurses pocket guide* (14th ed.). Philadelphia, PA: F.A. Davis.

Herdman, H., & Kamitsuru, S. (2014). *NANDA International, Inc. Nursing diagnoses: Definitions & classification 2015–2017* (10th ed.). Wiley Blackwell. Retrieved on November 2016 from: http://iaud.ac.ir

Hockenberry, M., & Wilson, D. (2013). *Wong's essentials of pediatric nursing* (9th ed.). St. Louis, MO: Elsevier-Mosby.

Hockenberry, M., & Wilson, D. (2015). *Wong's nursing care of infants and children* (10th ed.). St. Louis, MO: Elsevier-Mosby.

Jalil, E. R. (2016). *NANDA nursing diagnosis list 2015–2017*. Retrieved on November 2016 from: http://health-conditions.com/nanda-nursing-diagnosis-list-2015-2017/

Kyle, T., & Carman, S. (2017). *Essentials of pediatric nursing* (3rd ed.). Philadelphia, PA: Lippincott Williams & Wilkins.

Pillitteri, A. (2014). *Maternal and child health nursing* (7th ed.). New York: Lippincott Williams & Wilkins.

Chapter 11

Psychiatric diagnoses

Just the facts

In this chapter, you'll learn:

♦ nursing diagnoses that correlate with common psychiatric medical diagnoses.

A look at psychiatric diagnoses

This chapter covers common psychiatric medical diagnoses. Each entry provides a list of a few of the major nursing diagnoses and related factors to be considered after your assessment of a patient with the particular medical diagnosis. Remember that the nursing diagnoses listed here represent the needs most commonly associated with the medical condition; however, your patient may have different needs.

Abusive disorders, sexual or physical

- Dysfunctional family processes related to violence
- Ineffective relationship related to history of domestic violence
- Posttrauma syndrome related to:
  - abandonment
  - interpersonal violence
    - physical neglect or abuse
    - sexual abuse or assault
    - experiencing dangerous events
- Risk for compromised human dignity related to abuse

Alcohol use disorder

- Anxiety related to:
  - alcohol withdrawal
  - poor self-concept
  - real or perceived threats to physical safety

- Chronic low self-esteem related to:
  - coping difficulties
  - guilt
  - shame about alcohol abuse
  - unmet expectations
- Dysfunctional family processes related to:
  - role disruptions caused by the patient's alcohol use disorder
  - ineffective family communication and coping
  - lack of life skills
  - refusal to obtain or accept help from others
- Imbalanced nutrition: Less than body requirements related to:
  - effects of chronic alcohol intake on digestive organs
  - interference of alcohol in absorption and metabolism of nutrients
  - poor dietary intake while consuming alcohol
- Insomnia related to:
  - alcohol use disorder and decreased rapid-eye-movement sleep cycle
  - alcohol decreasing total sleep time
  - alcohol-induced sleep disorders, especially sleep apnea
- Risk for injury related to:
  - alcohol withdrawal
  - depression
  - impaired judgment
  - seizures
  - sensory deficits
  - suicidal ideation
- Risk-prone health behavior related to alcohol use disorder
  - Negative emotionality in the family
  - Peer or parental addictive behaviors
  - Lack of individual resiliency

Alcohol addiction and abuse can lead to risk for injury related to withdrawal, depression, seizures, and suicidal ideation, to name just a few. Another reason to stay addicted to water. Cheers!

Hallucinogenic use disorder

- Insomnia related to:
- hallucinogen use or intoxication as evidenced by verbal complaints of sleeping inability, nightmares, or interrupted sleep
- intense periods of wakefulness and alertness causing intensification of perceptions
- Risk for injury related to:
  - impaired judgment and disorientation
  - poisoning by use of adulterated street drugs
- Risk-prone health behavior related to substance use
  - Influence of peer behaviors
  - Desire to experience a drug high

Substance use disorder

- Chronic low self-esteem related to perceived failures and lack of positive feedback
- Ineffective coping related to maladaptive reliance on alcohol and other drugs
- Powerlessness related to lack of control over psychoactive substance use

Stimulant use disorder

- Decreased cardiac output related to stimulant use
- Deficient knowledge (risks of stimulant use) related to denial of need for information
- Fear related to altered thought processes
- Imbalanced nutrition: Less than body requirements related to placing greater importance on drug use than on eating
- Impaired social interaction related to isolation associated with drug use
- Ineffective health maintenance related to the effects of stimulant dependence on self-esteem
- Insomnia related to stimulant use
- Risk for disturbed personal identity related to use of psychoactive agents
- Risk for imbalanced body temperature related to stimulant use
- Risk for other-directed violence related to:
  - difficulty processing and interpreting thoughts
  - sensory overload from stimulant use
- Risk-prone health behavior related to substance use disorder

Sedative, hypnotic, or anxiolytic use disorder

- Deficient knowledge (risks of substance use) related to inability to process or retain information while impaired and in denial
- Ineffective denial related to feelings of low self-esteem
- Risk for infection related to:
  - compromised immunity
  - high-risk behaviors
  - insufficient knowledge about disease
- Risk-prone health behavior related to substance use

Adjustment disorder

- Complicated grieving related to:
  - inhibited grieving
  - multiple losses and bereavement processes
- Defensive coping related to:
  - inadequate support systems
  - personal vulnerability

  - ○ unmet expectations
  - ○ work overload and multiple stressors
- Impaired social interaction related to decreased perception of appropriate social behavior
- Risk-prone health behavior related to:
  - ○ disability requiring lifestyle changes
  - ○ impaired cognition
  - ○ inadequate support systems
  - ○ unresolved grieving

Anxiety disorder

- Anxiety related to:
  - ○ stresses in home or work environments
  - ○ disruptions in close interpersonal relationships
  - ○ threat to self-concept
  - ○ unmet needs
- Chronic low self-esteem related to lack of positive feelings and difficulty concentrating
- Imbalanced nutrition: Less than body requirements related to inability to ingest food due to psychological factors
- Social isolation related to panic state

Bipolar disorder

- Chronic low self-esteem related to depressive state and feelings of hopelessness, need to continue long-term medications
- Disturbed personal identity related to manic state
- Impaired home maintenance related to difficulty concentrating and flight of ideas
- Sleep deprivation related to manic state
- Risk for self-directed injury related to increased impulsive and irrational behavior

Delusional disorder

- Impaired social interaction related to delusional behavior
- Social isolation related to delusional behavior

Depression

- Chronic low self-esteem related to stress or loss
- Deficient diversional activity related to lack of interest
- Disturbed body image related to illness
- Imbalanced nutrition: More than/less than body requirements related to poor eating habits
- Ineffective coping related to obsessive negative thoughts and feelings

- Risk for caregiver role strain related to psychological needs of care recipient
- Risk for disturbed personal identity related to depressive state
- Risk for loneliness related to self-imposed social isolation
- Risk for self-directed violence related to lack of self-esteem and emotional pain
- Social isolation related to inability to engage in satisfying personal relationships

Dissociative disorder

- Disturbed personal identity related to underdeveloped ego, threat to self-concept, or childhood abuse or trauma
- Ineffective coping related to a severe level of repressed anxiety
- Interrupted family processes related to shift in health status of family member
- Risk for chronic low self-esteem related to perceived lack of belonging

Preoccupation with eating behaviors or rituals can lead to impaired social interaction.

Eating disorders

- Deficient knowledge (nutrition and eating disorders) related to lack of interest in learning
- Disturbed body image related to misperceived physical appearance
- Imbalanced nutrition: Less than body requirements related to:
  - excessive physical exercise
  - purging activities
  - refusal to eat
- Impaired social interaction related to withdrawal from peer group, fear of rejection, and preoccupation with eating behaviors or rituals
- Ineffective denial related to a lack of knowledge about real or potential dangers associated with eating disorders
- Ineffective impulse control related to disturbed body image
- Interrupted family processes related to a perfectionistic, overprotective, or chaotic family system

Gender dysphoria

- Anxiety related to conflict between desires and expected sex role behavior
- Disturbed personal identity related to conflict between anatomical sex and gender identity
- Ineffective sexuality pattern related to conflicts with sexual orientation
- Interrupted family processes related to family confusion and anxiety about gender of family member

Panic disorder
- Anxiety related to sudden attacks of fear or intense discomfort
- Chronic low self-esteem related to repeated episodes of apprehension and fear
- Posttrauma syndrome related to perception of adverse event or sudden loss

Personality disorder—Cluster A
- Impaired social interaction related to disorganized thinking, odd or eccentric behaviors, emotional coldness
- Ineffective coping related to:
  - inability to trust others
  - self-absorption
  - unusual perceptions and communication patterns
- Ineffective impulse control related to a lack of trust
- Interrupted family processes related to shift in physical or mental health status of family member

Personality disorder—Cluster B
- Impaired social interaction related to:
  - behaviors that produce hostility in others
  - inability to form healthy interpersonal relationships
  - low self-esteem
  - engaging in irresponsible or manipulative behavior
- Ineffective coping related to:
  - fear of abandonment
  - feelings of loneliness, emptiness, boredom
  - poor frustration tolerance
  - poor impulse control
- Ineffective impulse control related to seeking immediate gratification of personal needs
- Risk for other-directed or self-directed violence related to dramatic, emotional, or erratic behavior or low self-esteem

Personality disorder—Cluster C
- Anxiety related to a strong fear of nonacceptance or rejection
- Ineffective coping related to:
  - inability to ask for help
  - need to always be right and perfect
  - need to use rules and routines to maintain a secure environment
  - client's high level of sensitivity to criticism or disapproval
- Interrupted family processes related to rigidity in functions, roles, and rules

- Powerlessness related to:
  - ○ intellectualization or denial of feelings as a means to gain self-control
  - ○ perfectionistic behavior that protects against inferiority feelings
- Sleep deprivation related to prolonged psychological discomfort
- Social isolation related to an inability to establish and maintain relationships

Phobias

- Disturbed personal identity related to inability to have clarity about an object or situation
- Fear related to inability to identify probable causes
- Ineffective coping related to persistent irrational and disproportionate fear

Persistent irrational fear can lead to ineffective coping. Stand back, folks. I'm about to drop in for a visit.

Posttraumatic stress disorder

- Hopelessness related to feelings of helplessness and loss of control
- Posttrauma syndrome related to traumatic event
- Powerlessness related to uncertainty about the future, lack of sufficient coping skills, and support system

Schizophrenia

- Anxiety related to disturbance in thought process, perception, language, and communication
- Bathing self-care deficit related to apathy and delusions
- Caregiver role strain related to chronic illness

Sleep disorders

- Anxiety related to inability to sleep
- Insomnia related to:
  - ○ external factors, such as hospital routines, environmental noise, and changing work shifts
  - ○ medical illness
  - ○ pain
  - ○ psychological stress
  - ○ substance use
- Interrupted family processes related to family member not being able to fulfill role requirements because of lack of sleep

Patients with sleep disorders can experience anxiety related to inability to sleep. At this point, even the sheep have gone to sleep.

Somatoform and factitious disorders

- Bathing self-care deficit related to:
  - ○ activity intolerance
  - ○ neuromuscular or musculoskeletal impairment
  - ○ pain or discomfort
  - ○ perceptual or cognitive impairment

- Caregiver role strain related to unpredictable illness and conflict with care recipient
- Chronic pain related to unmet dependency needs or repressed anxiety as demonstrated by verbal complaints with no pathophysiological validation
- Deficient knowledge (healthful social interactions) related to:
  - denial
  - intense repressed anxiety level
  - lack of interest in learning
  - preoccupation with self and pain
- Disabled family coping related to struggle for control and power
- Disturbed body image related to low self-esteem evidenced by preoccupation with real or imagined altered body structure or function
- Ineffective coping related to:
  - extreme need for approval and acceptance
  - inability to manage emotional conflict
  - low self-esteem
  - unmet dependency needs
- Social isolation related to physical symptoms or disability

Vicarious traumatization

- Insomnia related to recurrent nightmares or dreams of personal death and fear of their recurrence
- Posttrauma syndrome related to the subjective experience of single or multiple traumatic events through repeated exposure to trauma victims (vicarious traumatization)
- Powerlessness related to:
  - inadequate problem-solving and coping skills
  - overwhelming anxiety

Selected references

American Psychiatric Association. (2013). *Diagnostic and statistical manual of mental disorders* (5th ed.). Arlington, VA: American Psychiatric Association.

Boyd, M. A. (2012). *Psychiatric nursing: Contemporary practice* (5th ed.). Philadelphia, PA: Lippincott Williams & Wilkins.

Halter, M. J., et al. (2014). *Varcarolis' foundations of psychiatric mental health nursing: A clinical approach* (7th ed.). St. Louis, MO: Saunders.

Mohr, W. K. (2013). *Psychiatric-mental health nursing: Evidence-based concepts, skills, and practices* (8th ed.). Philadelphia, PA: Lippincott Williams & Wilkins.

Varcarolis, E. M. (2015). *Manual of psychiatric nursing care planning: Assessment guides, diagnoses, psychopharmacology* (5th ed.). St. Louis, MO: Saunders.

Videbeck, S. L. (2014). *Psychiatric-mental health nursing* (6th ed.). Philadelphia, PA: Wolters Kluwer.

Appendix and index

NANDA nursing diagnosis list for 2018–2020

NANDA nursing diagnosis list— Domain 1: Health promotion

Class 1. Health awareness
- Decreased diversional activity engagement
- Readiness for enhanced health literacy
- Sedentary lifestyle

Class 2. Health management
- Frail elderly syndrome
- Risk for frail elderly syndrome
- Deficient community health
- Risk-prone health behavior
- Ineffective health maintenance
- Ineffective health management
- Readiness for enhanced health management
- Ineffective family health management
- Ineffective protection

NANDA nursing diagnosis list— Domain 2: Nutrition

Class 1. Ingestion
- Imbalanced nutrition: less than body requirements
- Readiness for enhanced nutrition
- Insufficient breast milk production
- Ineffective breastfeeding
- Interrupted breastfeeding
- Readiness for enhanced breastfeeding
- Ineffective adolescent eating dynamics
- Ineffective child eating dynamics
- Ineffective infant eating dynamics
- Ineffective infant feeding pattern
- Obesity
- Overweight
- Risk for overweight
- Impaired swallowing

Class 2. Digestion
None at present time

Class 3. Absorption
None at present time

Class 4. Metabolism
- Risk for unstable blood glucose level
- Neonatal hyperbilirubinemia
- Risk for neonatal hyperbilirubinemia
- Risk for impaired liver function
- Risk for metabolic imbalance syndrome

Class 5. Hydration
- Risk for electrolyte imbalance
- Risk for imbalanced fluid volume
- Deficient fluid volume
- Risk for deficient fluid volume
- Excess fluid volume

NANDA nursing diagnosis list— Domain 3: Elimination and exchange

Class 1. Urinary function
- Impaired urinary elimination
- Functional urinary incontinence
- Overflow urinary incontinence
- Reflex urinary incontinence
- Stress urinary incontinence
- Urge urinary incontinence
- Risk for urge urinary incontinence
- Urinary retention

Class 2. Gastrointestinal function
- Constipation
- Risk for constipation
- Perceived constipation
- Chronic functional constipation

- Risk for chronic functional constipation
- Diarrhea
- Dysfunctional gastrointestinal motility
- Risk for dysfunctional gastrointestinal motility
- Bowel incontinence

Class 3. Integumentary function

None at this time

Class 4. Respiratory function

- Impaired gas exchange

NANDA nursing diagnosis list— Domain 4: Activity/rest

Class 1. Sleep/rest

- Insomnia
- Sleep deprivation
- Readiness for enhanced sleep
- Disturbed sleep pattern

Class 2. Activity/exercise

- Risk for disuse syndrome
- Impaired bed mobility
- Impaired physical mobility
- Impaired wheelchair mobility
- Impaired sitting
- Impaired standing
- Impaired transfer ability
- Impaired walking

Class 3. Energy balance

- Imbalanced energy field
- Fatigue
- Wandering

Class 4. Cardiovascular/pulmonary responses

- Activity intolerance
- Risk for activity intolerance
- Ineffective breathing pattern
- Decreased cardiac output
- Risk for decreased cardiac output

- Impaired spontaneous ventilation
- Risk for unstable blood pressure
- Risk for decreased cardiac tissue perfusion
- Risk for ineffective cerebral tissue perfusion
- Ineffective peripheral tissue perfusion
- Risk for ineffective peripheral tissue perfusion
- Dysfunctional ventilatory weaning response

Class 5. Self-care

- Impaired home maintenance
- Bathing self-care deficit
- Dressing self-care deficit
- Feeding self-care deficit
- Toileting self-care deficit
- Readiness for enhanced self-care
- Self-neglect

NANDA nursing diagnosis list— Domain 5: Perception/cognition

Class 1. Attention

- Unilateral neglect

Class 2. Orientation

None at this time

Class 3. Sensation/perception

None at this time

Class 4. Cognition

- Acute confusion
- Risk for acute confusion
- Chronic confusion
- Labile emotional control
- Ineffective impulse control
- Deficient knowledge
- Readiness for enhanced knowledge
- Impaired memory

Class 5. Communication

- Readiness for enhanced communication
- Impaired verbal communication

NANDA nursing diagnosis list— Domain 6: Self-perception

Class 1. Self-concept
- Hopelessness
- Readiness for enhanced hope
- Risk for compromised human dignity
- Disturbed personal identity
- Risk for disturbed personal identity
- Readiness for enhanced self-concept

Class 2. Self-esteem
- Chronic low self-esteem
- Risk for chronic low self-esteem
- Situational low self-esteem
- Risk for situational low self-esteem

Class 3. Body image
- Disturbed body image

NANDA nursing diagnosis list— Domain 7: Role relationship

Class 1. Caregiving roles
- Caregiver role strain
- Risk for caregiver role strain
- Risk for impaired parenting
- Readiness for enhanced parenting

Class 2. Family relationships
- Risk for impaired attachment
- Dysfunctional family processes
- Interrupted family processes
- Readiness for enhanced family processes

Class 3. Role performance
- Ineffective relationship
- Risk for ineffective relationship
- Readiness for enhanced relationship
- Parental role conflict
- Ineffective role performance
- Impaired social interaction

NANDA nursing diagnosis list— Domain 8: Sexuality

Class 1. Sexual identity
None at present time

Class 2. Sexual function
- Sexual dysfunction
- Ineffective sexuality pattern

Class 3. Reproduction
- Ineffective childbearing process
- Risk for ineffective childbearing process
- Readiness for enhanced childbearing process
- Risk for disturbed maternal–fetal dyad

NANDA nursing diagnosis list— Domain 9: Coping/stress tolerance

Class 1. Post-trauma responses
- Risk for complicated immigration transition
- Post-trauma syndrome
- Risk for post-trauma syndrome
- Rape-trauma syndrome
- Relocation stress syndrome
- Risk for relocation stress syndrome

Class 2. Coping responses
- Ineffective activity planning
- Risk for ineffective activity planning
- Anxiety
- Defensive coping
- Ineffective coping
- Readiness for enhanced coping
- Ineffective community coping
- Readiness for enhanced community coping
- Compromised family coping
- Disabled family coping
- Readiness for enhanced family coping
- Death anxiety
- Ineffective denial
- Fear

- Grieving
- Complicated grieving
- Risk for complicated grieving
- Impaired mood regulation
- Readiness for enhanced power
- Impaired resilience
- Risk for impaired resilience
- Readiness for enhanced resilience
- Chronic sorrow
- Stress overload

Class 3. Neurobehavioral stress

- Acute substance withdrawal syndrome
- Risk for acute substance withdrawal syndrome
- Autonomic dysreflexia
- Risk for autonomic dysreflexia
- Decreased intracranial adaptive capacity
- Neonatal abstinence syndrome
- Disorganized infant behavior
- Risk for disorganized infant behavior
- Readiness for enhanced organized infant behavior

NANDA nursing diagnosis list—Domain 10: Life principles

Class 1. Values

None at this time

Class 2. Beliefs

- Readiness for enhanced spiritual well-being

Class 3. Value/belief/action congruence

- Readiness for enhanced decision-making
- Decisional conflict
- Impaired emancipated decision-making
- Risk for impaired emancipated decision-making
- Readiness for enhanced emancipated decision-making
- Moral distress
- Impaired religiosity
- Risk for impaired religiosity
- Readiness for enhanced religiosity
- Spiritual distress
- Risk for spiritual distress

NANDA nursing diagnosis list—Domain 11: Safety/protection

Class 1. Infection

- Risk for infection
- Risk for surgical site infection

Class 2. Physical injury

- Ineffective airway clearance
- Risk for aspiration
- Risk for bleeding
- Impaired dentition
- Risk for dry eye
- Risk for dry mouth
- Risk for falls
- Risk for corneal injury
- Risk for injury
- Risk for urinary tract injury
- Risk for perioperative positioning injury
- Risk for thermal injury
- Impaired oral mucous membrane integrity
- Risk for impaired oral mucous membrane integrity
- Risk for peripheral neurovascular dysfunction
- Risk for physical trauma
- Risk for vascular trauma
- Risk for pressure ulcer
- Risk for shock
- Impaired skin integrity
- Risk for impaired skin integrity
- Risk for sudden infant death
- Risk for suffocation
- Delayed surgical recovery
- Risk for delayed surgical recovery
- Impaired tissue integrity
- Risk for impaired tissue integrity
- Risk for venous thromboembolism

Class 3. Violence

- Risk for female genital mutilation
- Risk for other-directed violence
- Risk for self-directed violence
- Self-mutilation
- Risk for self-mutilation
- Risk for suicide

Class 4. Environmental hazards

- Contamination
- Risk for contamination
- Risk for occupational injury
- Risk for poisoning

Class 5. Defensive processes

- Risk for adverse reaction to iodinated contrast media
- Risk for allergic reaction
- Latex allergic reaction
- Risk for latex allergic reaction

Class 6. Thermoregulation

- Hyperthermia
- Hypothermia
- Risk for hypothermia
- Risk for perioperative hypothermia
- Ineffective thermoregulation
- Risk for ineffective thermoregulation

NANDA nursing diagnosis list— Domain 12: Comfort

Class 1. Physical comfort

- Impaired comfort

- Readiness for enhanced comfort
- Nausea
- Acute pain
- Chronic pain
- Chronic pain syndrome
- Labor pain

Class 2. Environmental comfort

- Impaired comfort
- Readiness for enhanced comfort

Class 3. Social comfort

- Impaired comfort
- Readiness for enhanced comfort
- Risk for loneliness
- Social isolation

NANDA nursing diagnosis list— Domain 13: Growth/development

Class 1. Growth

- None at present time

Class 2. Development

- Risk for delayed development

Index

Note: Page numbers followed by *f* and *t* indicate figures and tables, respectively.

Note: Page numbers followed by *f* and t indicate figures and tables, respectively.

Note: Page numbers followed by *f* and t indicate figures and tables, respectively.

Note: Page numbers followed by *f* and *t* indicate figures and tables, respectively.

Note: Page numbers followed by f and t indicate figures and tables, respectively.

Note: Page numbers followed by f and t indicate figures and tables, respectively.